Guide to Psychoactive Drugs:
An Up-to-the-Minute
Reference to
Mind-Altering Substances

About the Authors

RICHARD SEYMOUR, MA, is director of training and education for the Haight Ashbury Free Medical Clinics in San Francisco, California, and research and writing associate of founder and medical director David E. Smith, MD. In addition, he is the Clinics' historian and coordinator of funding and public relations. He also teaches courses in chemical dependency and addiction at Sonoma State University, John F. Kennedy University and San Francisco City College. In the turbulent early 1970s, he served as the clinics' executive administrator.

Seymour was the first chairman of a statewide California coalition of drug abuse treatment programs and currently serves on both the Marin County Drug Abuse Advisory Board and the California Alcoholism and Drug Counselors Education Program. He has been instrumental in the development of physician- and nurse-training courses in drug abuse diagnosis and treatment, prevention, and proper prescribing practices. As an international consultant, Seymour is currently developing a world symposium on cultural approaches to substance abuse. A prolific author, he has written many articles and treatment protocols on drug abuse, as well as four novels, short stories and two volumes of poetry. With Dr. Smith, he edits *Addictions Alert*, a monthly national newsletter on advances in diagnosing and treating addictive disease. Recent books include: *The Little Black Pill Book*, *The Coke Book*, *MDMA*, *Drugfree*, and *The Haight Ashbury Free Medical Clinics: Still Free After All These Years*.

DAVID E. SMITH, MD, is president and medical director of the Haight Ashbury Free Medical Clinics, which he founded in 1967. He is also associate clinical professor of toxicology, Department of Pharmacology, University of California Medical School at San Francisco. One of the nation's foremost experts on drugs and drug abuse, Dr. Smith has been a consultant to numerous government agencies and medical and health professionals. A pioneer in the development of addictionology as a medical subspecialty, his first priority remains treating destitute drug abusers in Haight Ashbury.

Dr. Smith and his colleagues have done seminal research on many facets of drug abuse. The treatment protocols he has developed for stimulants, sedative-hypnotics, PCP and other drugs are now used throughout the world. Recent programs developed by Dr. Smith include treatment and support for addicted physicians and nurses, and a system of cocaine recovery support groups.

Founder and editor of the *Journal of Psychoactive Drugs*, and editor with Richard Seymour of *Addictions Alert*, Dr. Smith serves on the editorial boards of several professional journals and has written and edited numerous books and articles. These include: *PCP: Problems and Prevention*, *Amphetamine Use, Misuse and Abuse*, *Drugs in the Classroom*, *Barbiturates: Their Use, Misuse and Abuse*, *A Multicultural View of Drug Abuse*, and *Substance Abuse in the Workplace*.

Guide to Psychoactive Drugs: An Up-to-the-Minute Reference to Mind-Altering Substances

Richard B. Seymour, MA and David E. Smith, MD

Harrington Park Press
New York • London

0-918393-43-4

Published by
Harrington Park Press, Inc., 12 West 32 Street, New York, New York 10001

EUROSPAN/Harrington, 3 Henrietta Street, London WC2E 8LU England

Harrington Park Press, Inc., is a subsidiary of The Haworth Press, Inc., 12 West 32 Street, New York, New York 10001.

Guide to Psychoactive Drugs: An Up-to-the-Minute Reference to Mind-Altering Substances was originally published as *The Physician's Guide to Psychoactive Drugs* in 1987 by The Haworth Press, Inc.

Cover design by Marshall Andrews.

Library of Congress Cataloging-in-Publication Data

Seymour, Richard, 1937-
    The physician's guide to psychoactive drugs.

    Bibliography: p.
    Includes index.
    1. Psychotropic drugs. 2. Psychopharmacology. 3. Substance abuse. I. Smith, David E. (David Elvin), 1939- . II. Title. [DNLM: 1. Psychotropic Drugs. 2. Substance Abuse. QV 77 S521p]
RM316.S49   1987   615'.788   87-354
ISBN 0-918393-43-4

CONTENTS

Introduction

The wonders of modern science and the wisdom of ancient times have brought us a bewildering variety of chemicals that effect the human mind. A number of these chemicals cause, in some way, effects that are considered desirable by the people who make use of them in nonmedical ways. These are the substances that we refer to as psychoactive drugs.

There are a great many such drugs, and more are being discovered, invented, or synthesized all the time, but basically they can be organized into four categories:

- Narcotics/analgesics
- Central nervous system depressants
- Central nervous system stimulants
- Psychedelics/psychotomimetics/hallucinogenics

These categories are not always clearly defined. For example, nearly all psychoactive drugs can have some psychedelic (change-of-consciousness) effects, and some drugs, such as the methoxylated amphetamines, may have the properties of two different categories. However, the properties and effects of the substances in each category are similar, so the general orientation they provide may aid us in understanding the overall scheme—the broad picture of these substances and of the people who use, misuse, or abuse them.

The first section of this book is devoted to the four categories of these psychoactive, affecting-the-psyche, or central nervous system (CNS) drugs. For each category there is a general introduction that includes the overall history of the drug group and detailed information on treatment that pertains to the group as a whole. Although this book is not intended to be a treatment manual, these introductions provide both the layperson and the health professional with some idea of what treatment with psychoactive drugs entails.

After the introduction, each category contains sections on the individual drugs within the broader group. Each of these contains enough information on the specific drugs to provide a quick reference about their nature, appearance, use, and dangers, and about their use in treatment. The reader can then refer on to the categoric introduction for further information.

The second section of the book contains a series of short essays on different aspects of substance abuse and substance abuse treatment that are common to all four categories. These discussions include information on treatment facilities, ways in which users manipulate prescribers to get drugs, and medical complications of drug use.

In general, this book is intended to provide up-to-date and understandable information about psychoactive drugs and their use for anyone who needs it.

SECTION ONE: THE NATURE OF PSYCHOACTIVE DRUGS

Narcotics/Analgesics

HISTORICAL PERSPECTIVE

The term "narcotic" is derived from the Greek *narkotikos*, which means numbness or stupor. In general, it means any drug that produces sleep, lethargy, and the relief of pain. Originally, the term referred to opium and to any drug derived from opium, such as heroin, morphine, or codeine.

Some confusion is created by the enforcement community's practice of referring to any potent illegal drug as a narcotic, including the stimulant cocaine. Although federal law classifies the coca leaf and cocaine as narcotics, we will follow the medical definitions and place these drugs among the central nervous system stimulants where they belong.

These drugs are also called analgesics because of their ability to suppress pain. The overall class of drugs includes opiates (drugs derived from opium) and opiodes (synthetic drugs that have similar effects).

Natural opiates are all derived from preparations extracted from the opium poppy bulb. The crudest of these is opium itself, which is boiled down from the sap bled from the poppy seed bulbs in much the way that maple syrup and maple sugar are produced from the sap of the maple tree. In this process, the bulbs are cut and bled soon after the poppy petals have matured and fallen away. The boiled raw opium is dark, resinous, and often tarlike in appearance, and it may give off a flowery odor.

In eastern countries, this resin itself is often smoked for its sedative, euphoriant, and hallucinogenic qualities. In the West, more refined forms are usually used, both as pharmaceuticals and as street drugs.

Although some other drugs have similar antiquity of use for religious purposes, opium and its products are among the oldest drugs still in use in the practice of medicine. The history of this drug is extensive.

The opium poppy, *Papaver somniferum*, originated in Asia Minor. It is referred to in a six-thousand-year-old Sumerian tablet as the "joy plant," and it appears in a sculpture from the same period as well as in Egyptian pictography. Both Virgil and Ovid refer to its properties. Representations of the Greek and Roman gods of sleep, Hypnos and Somnos, show them either wearing or carrying poppies.

Opium was well known to Classical Greek physicians, who ground the entire plant or used opium extract. The Greek physician Galen listed the medical indications of this drug in his practice, saying it:

> . . . resists poison and venomous bites, cures chronic headache, vertigo, deafness, epilepsy, apoplexy, dimness of sight, loss of voice, asthma, coughs of all kinds, spitting of blood, tightness of breath, colic, the lilac poison, jaundice, hardness of the spleen stone, urinary complaints, fever, dropsies, leprosies, the trouble to which women are subject, melancholy and all pestilences. (Smith and Gay, 1972)

Although the use of opium in medicine was lost to the West after the fall of Rome, the Arab world retained knowledge of it. In fact, owing to the Muslim injunctions against the use of alcohol, opium was used extensively in the Arab world as a recreational drug. Its medical use was regained in Europe during the Renaissance when the works of Galen and the Moorish physician Avicenna became the standard texts for medical education.

Many people have a mistaken notion that opium originated in China. Actually, the spread of opium abuse in China did not occur until the latter part of the 18th century. At that time, Portuguese, English, and American traders, with government backing, established a lucrative trade in the drug. The Chinese government resisted, and a series of engagements were fought with the British that came to be known as the Opium Wars. The British won, and the settlement resulted in the establishment of Hong Kong as a British Crown Colony and the payment of twenty-one million dollars by China as reparation for destroyed opium.

In medicine, opiates are used primarily for their analgesic (pain-killing) and constipating effects. The effects of these drugs vary both by the dosage and by the degree of refinement and purity of the particular preparation. Because they are constipating, low-grade opiates are used to treat diarrhea.

As street drugs, opiates are prized for their production of euphoria and feelings of well-being. The "rush" that usually comes on when the drug is injected has been compared by some users to a total-body sexual orgasm. These drugs also have antipsychotic, sedative, and relaxant qualities and are often used in a drug cycle to counter the more unpleasant effects of long-term stimulant abuse.

The drug group includes natural opium alkaloids; synthetic derivatives of opiates, synthetic opiatelike drugs, and synthetic opiatelike drugs of low addiction liability and low potency. Sometimes narcotic antagonists are included on the list because they bind to similar sites in the brain even though they have no narcotic effects. All these drugs act by attaching to receptor sites in the central nervous system and producing chemical changes within the brain itself. Research in the past decade has shown that under normal conditions, and when stimulated by such diverse means as acupuncture and aerobic exercise such as running, the body produces its own internal opiatelike substances. These substances are called endorphins. They attach to many of the same receptor sites as narcotics and have similar effects. It is these endorphins that cause euphoric feelings after exercise, cessation of pain following minor injuries, and shock symptoms in trauma. Pain, of course, is the prime stimulant for the production of endorphins.

Several occurrences in the 19th century contributed both to the medical usefulness of opiates and to their abuse potential. In 1806, Frederich Seturner isolated morphine, the primary active ingredient in opium. Development of the hypodermic syringe in 1853 made it possible to deliver this purer drug form quickly into the body for rapid relief of pain or onset of euphoria with a rush. Finally, in 1874, C. R. Wright synthesized diacety morphine using refined morphine and acetic anhydride. This substance was first marketed by Bayer Pharmaceutical Products of Elberfeld, Germany, in 1898 under the trade name Heroin.

Morphine was used extensively as a painkiller for wounded troops during the American Civil War. After that war, morphine addiction among veterans was a national health problem. Opiates in general were often a prime ingredient in a variety of tonics and elixirs used mainly by women. At the turn of the century, it could be said that the average opiate abuser was a middle-aged, middle-class white housewife and mother.

Two opiate preparations in common use at the turn of the century were favored by many artists and writers. These were paregoric, a dilute tincture of opium combined with camphor and used medically for diarrhea, and laudanum, a simple tincture of opium in alcohol. Both are still on the market.

The natural opiate in most general use today is codeine, combined with a variety of other ingredients. Codeine preparations usually come in pill form and are often prescribed for dental postoperative pain and other moderate pain.

There are currently several hundred natural or synthetic narcotic analgesics on the market or being used illicitly. The following list, compiled by Kenneth Blum (1984), indicates the most prevalent of these by category:

- *Natural opium alkaloids*
  Morphine
  Codeine
- *Synthetic derivatives of opiates*
  Dihydromorphinone (Dilaudid®)
  Diacetylmorphine (heroin)
  Methyldihydromorphinone (metopon)
  Hydrocodone (Hycodan®)
- *Synthetic opiatelike drugs*
  Phenazocine (Prinadol®)
  Meperidine (Demerol®)
  Alphaprodine (Nisentil®)
  Anileridine (Leritine®)
  Piminodine (Alvodine®)
  Diphenoxylate (with atropine, as Lomotil®)
  Methadone (Dolophine®)
  Levorphanol (Levo-Dromoran®)
- *Synthetic opiatelike drugs of low addiction liability and potency*
  Propoxyphene (Darvon®)
  Ethoheptamine (Zactane®)
  Pentazocine (Talwin®)

NOTE: Not included in the list of opiatelike synthetics is fentanyl (with droperidol as Innovar), a narcotic analgesic that has given rise to a series of street-abused, high-potency analogues.

Public opinion regarding chemical dependency or addiction to narcotics was quite different in the 19th century from what it is today. There was no connotation of criminality or underworld connections. These drugs were readily available. Dependence on them tended to be viewed as a vice or as a personal misfortune but not as a crime.

The first law pertaining to opiates is thought to have been both racist and political in its motivation. It was an ordinance passed in the city of San Francisco in 1875 banning the smoking of opium by the city's Chinese. Several tax acts followed, but the national statute that criminalized recreational use of these drugs was the Harrison Narcotic Act of 1914.

Narcotic drugs can be ingested, injected either intravenously or intramuscularly, snorted, sipped, taken in pill or tablet form, or smoked. A method of use called "chasing the dragon" involves vaporizing the substance and then inhaling the vapor.

ACUTE AND CHRONIC TOXICITY

Narcotics mainly affect the brain and bowel. In the brain, they cause relief of pain, relaxation, and drowsiness; suppression of the cough center; and stimulation of the vomiting center. They can also cause mental clouding and inability to concentrate.

The desired effects in narcotic abuse include a rush that has been compared to sexual orgasm; it occurs when potent narcotic preparations are injected intravenously. Users cite feelings of euphoria, a melting of troubles—feelings that everything is all right and the user is in control.

These drugs are not reliable for sleep induction. Some people become anxious, restless, and wakeful after taking them, while others fall into a twilight sleep marked by vivid dreams.

Opiates cause the pupils of the eyes to contract, sometimes to pinpoints. They can cause profuse and uncomfortable sweating. With large dosages, nausea, vomiting, and depression of breathing can take place.

Most postoperative and other patients who must take these drugs for pain find the experience singularly unpleasant and are relieved when their pain has subsided to where they no longer need to be used. For some, however, the narcotics produce a compulsion to continue use, even before the onset of physical dependence.

Sufferers from chronic pain may also develop a dependence on opiates as the only means of dealing with their pain. One unfortunate aspect of this situation is that in many areas chronic pain victims are lumped in with opiate addicts and considered to be drug abusers. Chronic pain is perhaps one of the more troublesome medical problems we have today from a philosophic and treatment standpoint.

In our culture, the drug of choice for the majority of opiate street abusers is heroin. Most of these heroin abusers started out as recreational users, not as postoperative patients or chronic pain victims. The heroin used tends to be of a low purity, 4% to 6%, and is injected.

Acute toxicity is usually the result of an overdose. The user either takes too much of the drug or inadvertently buys an unusually potent formulation. In either case, the patient becomes comatose and cyanotic, with slow respiration and pinpointed pupils.

Chronic toxicity is associated with opiate or opioid dependence. Dependence can occur with any opium derivative or synthetic narcotic, as can an overdose. Prolonged use of these drugs usually results in physical dependence, marked by withdrawal symptomatology if use is terminated, and in tolerance, wherein the victim needs an ever increasing amount of the drug to achieve any desired effects.

Treatment of Acute Toxicity: Overdose

Fortunately, overdose with either an opiate or an opioid can be reversed by administration of the narcotic antagonist naloxone (Narcan®). This is usually done in the emergency unit. The antagonist should be injected intravenously, with 0.2 to 0.8 mg given initially. If the patient is in shock and has low blood pressure, 1.0 mg of the antagonist can be injected sublingually at the beginning and the injection repeated sublingually or intravenously to gain a response. The sublingual injection site must be carefully watched for oozing blood, which may be aspirated and may cause serious consequences.

In opiate or opioid overdose, pupillary dilation and an elevation in the level of consciousness will occur within 20 seconds to 1 minute following intravenous administration of naloxone. If this response is obtained, a second injection of naloxone, 0.2 mg intravenously, should follow for prolonged effect. If the overdose was caused by methadone or propoxyphene napsylate (Darvon®), however, both long-acting narcotics, repeated doses of naloxone will be required every 1 to 2 hours. (Naloxone is a short-acting narcotic antagonist, and the opiate effect of long-acting narcotics will outlast the antagonist effect of a single dose.)

Ancillary treatment is similar to that used for shock. It should be provided while the client is being taken to emergency or wherever the antagonist is available, and these measures should continue throughout antagonist treatment. These general supportive measures include clearing the airway, maintaining respiration through such means as cardiopulmonary resuscitation (CPR) or artificial respiration, keeping the patient warm, and elevating the feet. The similarity between symptoms of shock and those of narcotic overdose has led some investigators to the supposition that the cause of shock may be produced by an overdose—that is, an overproduction—of those internal opioids, endorphins.

Narcotic overdoses usually indicate a long-term abuse pattern or narcotic addiction. Therefore, the patient should be counseled and if possible referred for long-range treatment.

Treatment for Chronic Toxicity: Dependence

A wide variety of modalities are available for treating opiate and opioid dependence. At one end of the scale is maintenance. Essentially, this is not treatment at all, but merely the providing of the drug of choice or substitution of what is considered a more desirable alternative. In Great Britain and certain other countries, some users are provided with clinical doses of heroin itself, although the British have shifted to methadone maintenance in about 85% of patients. In the United States, the long-acting narcotic methadone is used. Proponents of methadone mainte-nance point out that this drug can be administered orally, and the long-term effectiveness facilitates daily administration. At the very least, it provides narcotic-dependent individuals who have been unable to detox-ify with a means of leading a relatively normal life. Opponents point out that methadone detoxification takes longer than heroin detoxification, and methadone dependence is more difficult to treat than heroin depen-dence.

A much less controversial use of methadone is in detoxification. Its use is similar to the phenobarbital substitution and withdrawal used in treat-ment of sedative-hypnotic dependence. Methadone is substituted for the opiate on which the patient is dependent. The methadone dosage during the first 2 days is usually 10 to 40 mg. This is followed by a gradual dosage reduction over a 3 to 21-day period or until the patient is drug free. This form of detoxification usually requires hospitalization.

Non-narcotic symptomatic medication may be used on an outpatient basis to relieve the symptoms of narcotic withdrawal. This practice usu-ally includes the use of a sedative, a hypnotic, and an antispasmodic for relief of anxiety, insomnia, and gastrointestinal upset, respectively.

Acupuncture and other nondrug approaches have been used with vary-ing degrees of success. Withdrawal from narcotics may be uncomforta-ble, even painful, but it is not in itself dangerous or life threatening. Many treatment modalities make no use of any ameliorative medical pro-cedures in the withdrawal process. These may rely on strong religious belief, ongoing counseling and various sociopsychologic therapy tech-niques, peer pressure and support, or sheer intimidation to gain results.

Some programs totally isolate the patient from society to provide a *nurturing* and *safe* environment for recovery. Some of these programs have had excellent results as far as they go, but often the patient ends up transferring dependence from the drug to the program.

DEPENDENCE-RELATED MEDICAL PROBLEMS

Overdose and dependence are not the only problems one encounters with narcotic users. When heroin finally reaches the user, for example, it may be cut with a variety of substances, including starch, quinine, baking soda, and mannitol. Some cuts may have deleterious effects of their own that should be taken into consideration.

Nonsterile needles and other paraphernalia, contaminated drugs, and the sharing of needles can lead to a variety of problems. These include needle abscesses, bacterial infections, hepatitis, and acquired immune deficiency syndrome (AIDS). Hepatitis is probably the most frequent complication of heroin abuse. While rarely fatal if diagnosed and treated, this disease can cause great damage to the liver and other internal organs. Bacterial infection of the heart occurs quite often and is more often fatal than hepatitis. Other infections can cause acute pulmonary congestion and edema.

By far the most deadly current complication of needle use in drug abuse is AIDS. Although the spread of this disease through needle-using populations can be stopped by sterilization and nonsharing, this group still represents the second highest rate of AIDS victims. The tragedy here is that it is so unnecessary. Nationwide educational and informational campaigns are in progress to stop the spread of AIDS in this population. The message is simple and direct: "Don't share a needle with *anyone.*"

ALPHA METHYL FENTANYL

Category: Schedule I

Product names: None

Street names: China white, fentanyl, synthetic heroin, AMF

Description: A yellowish white crystalline powder sold in the same manner as Persian heroin, i.e., in small aluminum-foil packets. Currently, the smallest amount sold, a "tenth," costs about $100. A tenth is said to contain enough for 20 to 30 doses for the nonaddicted user. This is about 0.01 to 0.05 mg per dose compared to a national average of 8 to 16 mg per dose of street heroin. Single-dose packets costing $5.00 each have been reported (Henderson, 1982).

Means of ingestion: Intravenous injection

General Information

Alpha methyl fentanyl (AMF) is an analogue of fentanyl, an analgesic (pain-killing) drug similar to morphine and used in hospitals under the brand names Lunovar® and Sublimaze®. Alpha methyl fentanyl may be 1000 times more potent than morphine. Obviously a powerful pain killer, AMF is but one of a nearly limitless series of easily synthesized narcotic analgesics. Some of its effects are similar to those of heroin, but AMF is not an opiate. It is a fully synthetic narcotic. Pharmaceutical fentanyl, by itself, is a controlled drug, administered by health professionals who can accurately control dosages. Its analogues, i.e., drugs like the original but with minor chemical changes, are not controlled. New ones could be developed as rapidly as the current ones could be made illegal. The implications of an ongoing chain of quasi-legal, easily manufactured "synthetic heroins" are an enforcement nightmare.

Sold as a drug of deception for heroin, or mixed with heroin, AMF is undetectable by standard lab tests for opiates. Clandestine laboratories producing analogues of fentanyl can eliminate the French, Southeast Asian, or any other overseas connection, making current enforcement efforts against the international narcotics trade both meaningless and useless. The use of these drugs is following "Persian" heroin into a middle-class white market that has little or no experience with opiates.

In December of 1980, the fentanyl analogue appeared on the street in New York City. By January, it had appeared in San Francisco and Los Angeles as well. Billed as "China white," after a powerful and perhaps legendary strain of heroin from Southeast Asia, it is usually recognized by users as not being heroin, at least when sold in pure form.

Fentanyl travels directly to the brain after intravenous injection and binds to the μ (*mu*) receptor, one of the several opiate receptors occupied by heroin and morphine. Onset of action is very rapid, and the effects last from 30 to 60 minutes (Ayers et al., 1981). While most AMF is sold as heroin, a growing number of habitual users know generally what it is and refer to it as "synthetic." Tests for its presence have been developed but are not generally available.

Dangers

Because of the strength of fentanyl analogues, there is great danger of overdose and death. This danger is especially great when they are sold as drugs of deception or mixed with street heroin to "give it more pep." Like other misrepresented drugs, AMF analogues may cause confusion in treatment centers where even the slightest delay in diagnosis can be fatal. Fluctuation in strength makes accurate "safe" dosages difficult for users to ascertain. Although a lab test has been developed, the presence of fentanyl in the body is still difficult to establish through tests of urine, feces, saliva, or blood.

Fentanyl itself is a powerful synthetic narcotic-analgesic, legitimately manufactured in the United States. Because of its rapid onset of action and short duration, it is used in obstetric anesthesia. Addiction to fentanyl can occur, but we have seen this addiction primarily in health professionals. AMF is about ten times more potent than clinical fentanyl. Because of this potency, China white produced a number of overdose deaths in California and demonstrated a high level of addiction in the drug culture. AMF is a chemical that is not manufactured legitimately but is synthesized in illicit laboratories, demonstrating that such labs have a much higher level of technical skill in synthesizing drugs than previously thought.

Emergency Treatment

Fentanyl overdose patients must be given immediate treatment including cardiopulmonary resuscitation (CPR), artificial respiration, and the administration of a narcotic antagonist such as naloxone. The preferred route of initial administration of naloxone is intravenous. The line between coma and death is very narrow.

Long-term Treatment

Addiction to fentanyl should be managed like any other narcotic dependence, with appropriate medication for detoxification and an aftercare program to prevent relapse. Because of its potency, AMF withdrawal can be more severe on a dose-equivalent basis than heroin withdrawal, but qualitatively it should be managed the same way.

HEROIN

Chemical name: Diacetylmorphine

Category: Schedule I

Product names: None in the United States. Diacetylmorphone elsewhere.

Street names: Big H, boy, brown sugar, caballo, chiva, crap, doo-jee, estuffa, scag, smack, stofa, stuff

Description: Usually a powder. May range in color from white to gray or dark brown. Some preparations are gray-and-white streaked or pink. Street heroin is usually cut with a variety of substances and runs well under 10% in strength. In recent years, much more potent heroin at comparatively high prices has been available from the Near East, the Far East, and Mexico.

Means of ingestion: Heroin is usually injected either subcutaneously, intramuscularly, or directly into a vein. Injection will maximize efficient use of the drug and produce the rush effect, highly prized by users. The appearance of higher potency heroin has led to smoking, or "chasing the dragon," often in a pattern with cocaine freebasing.

General Information

Heroin (diacetylmorphine) was first synthesized in 1874 by the English research chemist C. R. Wright, using refined morphine and acetic anhydride. Twenty years later, German researchers found that this substance had some success in the treatment of a variety of respiratory ailments and could also be used as a "nonaddicting" substitute for morphine and codeine. In 1898, Bayer Pharmaceutical Products of Elberfeld, Germany, coined the brand-name Heroin and launched the drug on the international market (McCoy, 1972). For several years, heroin enjoyed a vogue as a cough medicine and general analgesic. On the basis of David Musto's research, John Morgan, MD, has pointed out in his lectures on addiction stereotypes that at the turn of the century the American heroin "addict" was a white, middle-aged, middle-class housewife with two or more children (Musto, 1973).

Soon, however, heroin became an increasingly notorious street drug among poor and minority populations. Within a few years, its medical use became restricted, and today in the United States it is totally illegal. Although the drug is still recognized in Great Britain as a potent medical analgesic, and even though much stronger specific painkillers are used in American hospitals, heroin has such a sinister reputation in this country that the few attempts made to legalize its use, even for research or highly specific treatment indications, are met with extreme political, law-enforcement, and popular objections.

National concern about heroin addiction heightened in the late 1960s when a nationwide "epidemic" of heroin use spread through the white, basically middle-class, counterculture. The incidence of heroin experimentation is considered to have fallen off in recent years. Long-term use, however, has remained fairly constant, with demographics indicating a progressively aging user population. In any event, heroin addiction is still a major national problem. At the Haight-Ashbury Free Medical Clinic's Drug Abuse Treatment, Rehabilitation and Aftercare Project, one of our chief drug-treatment concerns is still heroin addiction. Within the last few years, the abuse of heroin has spread to a whole new population: well-to-do overachievers who are smoking high purity "Persian" heroin from the Near East. This is often done in a pattern with the smoking of freebase cocaine.

Developments allied to heroin abuse include the use of fentanyl analogues such as the extremely potent alpha-methyl fentanyl, often called "China white" in reference to a mythical, high-potency form of heroin. A highly dangerous development is the recent outbreak of drug-induced parkinsonism, brain damage, and paralysis caused by the impurity MPTP in the meperidine (Demerol®) analogue MPPP.

Pure heroin is a white powder with a bitter taste. Street samples may vary in color from white to dark brown because of manufacturing impurities or additives. Most street heroin contains only 2 to 4% actual heroin. The rest of the powder may be composed of such fillers as sugars, starch, powdered milk, or quinine. An exception to this is the Persian heroin mentioned earlier, which may run as high as 92% purity.

Heroin can be smoked, snorted, or injected under the skin, into a muscle, or directly into a vein. The initial reaction to the drug is usually negative, and includes nausea, sweating, and a general feeling of discomfort. After a few doses, users report experiencing a rush of good feeling that lasts a few minutes, followed by drowsiness. The rush appears to be most intense when the drug is injected intravenously.

At this writing, there are several new and potent forms of heroin on the street. "Malaysian Pink" has been analyzed at about 50% heroin. This substance is dyed a bright pink as a street trademark. (As could be expected, some low-potency street heroin is now dyed the same way.) "Mexican Tar" looks like opium but runs about 37% heroin, and "Amsterdam Marble," which looks like gray-and-white marble, runs about 63% heroin. These extremely potent preparations carry a great risk of unintentional fatal overdose. The situation is complicated by the lookalikes and drugs of deception that are marketed to mimic a successful drug preparation. Thus, there can be a wildly fluctuating potency, and even content to drugs that look exactly alike.

Dangers

Heroin users run a high risk for tolerance, dependence, and addiction. A highly uncomfortable, though not life-threatening, physical withdrawal symptomatology occurs whenever the addicted user does not reapply the drug at regular intervals, or attempts to detoxify. Heroin can be physically, mentally, and sexually debilitating. Often its use completely replaces sex in the user's life. The drug is also very, very expensive. Addicts are often forced into a life of crime to support their addiction. There is a great risk of fatal overdose. The needle user who shares needles is vulnerable to a variety of serum-spread diseases such as hepatitis and the still incurable Acquired Immune Deficiency Syndrome or AIDS. There is also the threat of needle abscesses and other infections.

Emergency Treatment

Overdoses can be treated with narcotic antagonists such as Narcan, which "kick" the opiate molecules out of their central nervous system receptor sites, blocking these sites. The reaction of a comatose overdose victim to these antagonists can be very dramatic. The victim should be-kept under observation until the opiate has been metabolized and the danger is over.

Long-term Treatment

There is a wide variety of detoxification and aftercare for heroin addicts. This includes "cold turkey" (any treatment that merely lets withdrawal run its course), outpatient counseling and non-narcotic medication, therapeutic communities or TCs, acupuncture, aerobic exercise, self-help groups such as Narcotics Anonymous, and methadone substitution and withdrawal. A course of treatment may depend on the individual's ability to withstand the withdrawal symptomatology, and this in turn may depend on the length, dosage level, and severity of the habit. In situations where all else has failed, methadone maintenance may be used.

Heroin addiction is often a long-term problem involving cyclic relapses. Return to use almost invariably leads back into full addiction. Even the use of pharmaceutical opiates may lead to a relapse. This makes management of pain for clean opiate addicts a difficult and sensitive issue. The recommended course is one of recovery through the adoption of a lifestyle that does not involve the use of any psychoactive substance, including alcohol.

METHADONE HYDROCHLORIDE

Chemical name: 4,4-diphenyl-6-dimethylamino-heptanone-3 hydrochloride

Category: Schedule II

Product names: Methadone, Dolophine®

Street names: None

Description: Methadone is a white crystalline material that is soluble in water. It is synthesized by Eli Lilly and Company and sold in liquid, tablet, and diskette form.

Means of ingestion: Injected, swallowed in pills, swallowed as diskettes, or mixed with drinkable substances such as orange juice. Note: While methadone itself is soluble in water, the diskettes are prepared in such a way as to make them insoluble. This is done to prevent their being dissolved and injected.

General Information

Methadone was first synthesized in Germany during World War II as a painkiller when Germany's access to raw opium, the basis of morphine and other opiate painkillers, was cut off. Although the chemical structure of methadone and heroin are quite different, their potencies as analgesics are similar, as is their pharmacologic profile in general (Blum, 1984).

Although methadone was developed as an analgesic, its primary use in the United States has been for the treatment of opiate addiction. In 1964, two New York physicians, Vincent Dole and Marie Nyswander, pioneers in addiction treatment research, proposed that methadone be used as a substitute for heroin in narcotic maintenance programs. England was using a system of providing heroin itself to addicts who enlisted with the National Health System for maintenance treatment. Dole and Nyswander selected methadone as their substitute agent because it was inexpensive, effective when taken orally — eliminating the need for injections — and of such prolonged duration, usually 36 to 48 hours, that daily administration on an outpatient basis was feasible (Unger, 1984). Also, it was theorized that since methadone was a synthetic manufactured under government licensing, it could be kept under control. By implication, so could the addicts who were using it.

The concept was that methadone would give addicts a more stable lifestyle and would minimize their illegal activities, such as stealing and hustling for money to pay for expensive street heroin. Methadone, provided daily at licensed clinics, would eliminate the pressure for buying heroin both by preventing opiate withdrawal symptoms and by blocking the euphoric action of opiates.

Unlike narcotic antagonists, which will block opiate receptor sites in the central nervous system and neutralize the effects of heroin, methadone does produce a "high" of its own. In maintenance, the dosage is controlled (titrated) to keep this opioid high at a minimum, just enough to reduce cravings for heroin or other opiates and to block or reduce the effects of other opiates such as heroin if the individual persists in injecting them. However, methadone will not block the effects of other nonopiate or opioid drugs such as alcohol, barbiturates, or cocaine.

Although methadone maintenance is often referred to in treatment circles as "a political solution to a medical problem," it is the treatment mode preferred by most heroin addicts themselves. In patients for whom all methods of detoxification have failed, methadone maintenance does at least provide a means to lead a relatively normal life, free from the criminal activity needed to support continuous narcotics addiction.

Dangers

The viability of methadone maintenance as a treatment modality has been a highly charged issue, argued and reargued in advisory committees and treatment-related agencies. Both sides in this continuing controversy list advantages and disadvantages. The primary disadvantage cited is that maintenance basically consists of trading one addiction for another – addiction, moreover, to a drug often considered to be more addictive and harder to detoxify from than heroin itself. Critics recall that one of the first uses of heroin was as a means of fighting morphine addiction. Many addicts seek treatment after only a short period of addiction to low-potency heroin in relatively low dosages. In these people, who have not yet developed a high tolerance, uninhibited assigning of maintenance may serve to solidify borderline addiction.

Increasing amounts of methadone are showing up in the illegal market. Again the memory that heroin was originally developed as a "nonaddicting" substitute for morphine and codeine cough medication comes back to haunt us. Many patients on maintenance supplement the miniscule methadone high with a large intake of alcohol or another sedative-hypnotic, or conversely with amphetamine or cocaine, none of which are diminished in effect by methadone's receptor-blocking action. (Mixing methadone with alcohol can result in severe liver damage.) There is a further danger that methadone may be used to replace alternative forms of treatment, just as it replaces heroin. Maintenance patients may receive their dose while missing out on counseling and other needed care.

Methadone can cause life-threatening overdoses. Chronic use can involve constipation, decreased sexuality, and other symptoms common to opiate addiction. Withdrawal is similar to heroin withdrawal, except that it lasts much longer.

In recent years, methadone maintenance has fallen into disfavor with virtually everyone but the maintenance clients themselves. While useful in certain extreme cases of opiate addiction, its general use in treatment does appear to have many drawbacks.

The employment of methadone as an agent to detoxify individuals addicted to heroin is much less controversial. Here the opiate-dependent individual is given methadone, usually on an outpatient basis, to block withdrawal effects, and then the methadone is gradually reduced over a 21-day period until the individual is referred to drug-free treatment. Methadone as a maintenance agent and methadone as a detoxification agent are two separate treatment strategies.

Emergency Treatment

Opiate overdoses, including methadone, can be treated with narcotic antagonists such as naloxone (Narcan®). With methadone or other long-acting synthetics, care must be taken to resupply the antagonist substance at regular intervals. Otherwise, the long-acting opioids will outlast antagonists in the system and reattach to the receptor sites, causing a lapse back into overdose.

Long-term Treatment

Withdrawal from methadone is similar to that from heroin. It is reported to be often longer and harder to attain. It is uncomfortable but not life threatening and can be accomplished by a variety of means. (See the section on heroin for an explication of these.)

MPPP

Chemical name: 1-methyl-4-phenyl-4-propionoxy-piperidine

Category: Schedule I

Product names: None

Street names: Sold as an analogue of meperidine (Demerol®), synthetic heroin, new heroin

Description: Usually described as brown, granular, and sticky, MPPP is an underground preparation used as an analogue of meperidine. Its appearance can vary as a drug of deception for heroin.

Means of ingestion: Injection

General Information

An illegally manufactured analogue of the painkiller meperidine (Demerol®), MPPP has the usual addictive and overdose problems associated with any opiate or opioid analgesic. Its greatest danger, however, comes from an often-present contaminant, MPTP. This contaminant, 1-methyl-4 phenyl-1,2,5,6, tetrahydropyridine (MPTP) is a by-product in the synthesis of 1-methyl-4-phenyl-4-propionoxy-piperidine (MPPP). MPTP is also a commercially available compound sold as a chemical intermediate (not a drug) by a number of industrial chemical companies (Langston et al., 1983). Since this substance is not meant for human consumption, its effects on animals or man have never been scientifically or systemically investigated.

The presence of MPTP in street compounds of the meperidine analogue MPPP seems to be the result of sloppy synthesis. A case report published in 1979 indicates that similar symptoms resulted from a botched synthesis of a meperidine analogue in the mid-1970s. In that case, the patient attempted to synthesize 4-pro-pyloxy-4-phenyl-N-methylpiperidine (PPMP) and took "short cuts." The patient reduced reaction time and used higher reaction temperatures, as well as neglecting to isolate and properly crystallize the resulting chemical. As a result, he got 4 hydroxy4-phenyl-N-methylpiperidine (HPMP). After shooting up a portion of it, he suffered parkinsonian paralysis characterized by the inability to speak, severe body rigidity, weakness, flat facial expression, and sensory confusion (Davis et al., 1979).

For all intents and purposes, MPTP is a contaminant in an illegally synthesized "synthetic heroin" related to meperidine. Meperidine itself is a synthetic painkiller used to reduce the moderate to severe pain of migraine headaches and childbirth. It is produced both under its generic name and also as Demerol and Pethadol. All precautions that apply to opiates apply to meperidine. In the street it is known as "cubes." It is also combined with aspirin, acetaminophen, caffeine, phenacetin, or promethazine and sold under various brand names for relief of mild to moderate pain. We want to emphasize that MPTP is *not* an ingredient in legitimate meperidine; it is a by-product found in drugs of deception that are clandestinely manufactured and sold on the street as "synthetic heroin."

Dangers

In early 1982, cases of severe parkinsonism began to surface in Northern California. By the beginning of July, MPTP and MPPP had been identified in samples of "new heroin" used by some of the victims. Researchers at the National Institute on Mental Health in Bethesda, Maryland, confirmed clinical suspicions that the new heroin might be causing the problem when they produced parkinsonism in monkeys by injecting them with a form of MPTP (Burns et al., 1983).

It is now fairly certain that use of the MPPP form of meperidine (Demerol®), contaminated with MPTP and sold as synthetic heroin, can cause permanent Parkinson's Disease symptoms by affecting the neurotransmitters in a specific area of the brain. At this writing, over 150 people in the San Francisco Bay Area are known to be affected, and cases are appearing in other parts of the country. There are probably many other victims who have not yet been identified.

Symptoms may be noted anywhere from 48 hours to 6 weeks after use of the contaminated drug. Early symptoms are stiffness of movement (almost arthritis), tremors, and in some cases, seizures. Symptoms may progress all the way to total paralysis. Paralysis has been so complete in some instances that the victims could respond to questions only by eye movement. The brain damage is irreversible. This "bad dope" can lead to permanent disability and paralysis.

The contaminated drug has been described as brown, granular, and sticky, but this description is not reliable, since its appearance may vary, making it almost impossible for the user to detect reliably. Victims have reported a burning sensation during injection, but there is no sure way of identifying the contaminated material short of careful laboratory analysis.

Emergency Treatment

There really is none. Anyone who has used the so-called synthetic or new heroin and is showing any of the above symptoms, should get to a treatment center immediately, if possible with a sample of the dope he or she has been taking.

Long-term Treatment

Paradoxically, MPTP and its victims are providing the first real breakthrough on the understanding and possibly the eventual cure of Parkinson's disease. Researchers are carefully studying the effects and mechanism of action of MPTP, with the suspicion that the cell death that occurs in Parkinson's disease may be caused by a natural substance in the body similar to MPTP.

Patients have responded to therapy with a combination of L-dopa and carbidopa (Sinemet®), used in treatment of conventional Parkinson's disease. These medications themselves can have side effects which limit their use and sometimes limit the treatment to temporary relief of symptoms.

PERSIAN HEROIN

Category: Schedule I

Product names: None

Street names: Persian brown, Persian, lemon dope, rufus, dava, Southwest Asian heroin

Description: Persian heroin is a dark reddish brown, granular powder. Unlike most street heroin, which is sold in "bags" (rubber balloons filled with 200 to 400 mg of powder) or as "spoons" (four bags or 1.0 to 1.5 g), Persian is usually sold in aluminum foil or waxed paper folded to form a small envelope. A single hit (25 mg) can be bought individually. The basic unit is the "tenth" (one-tenth of a gram or 100 mg), which sells for about $75.00. This compares to the greater bulk of the usual 2 to 4% street heroin dosage (approximately 100 to 200 mg), which generally runs to about $25.00 to $30.00.

Means of ingestion: Persian heroin can be injected, but it is usually insufflated (snorted) or smoked alone or mixed with marijuana or tobacco. Persian can also be taken orally, sublingually, or anally.

General Information

Heroin is a semisynthetic narcotic derived from morphine, the primary alkaloid found in opium. It produces euphoria and has analgesic (painkilling) effects. It reduces hunger and aggressive drives and, with long-term use, sexual drive and performance. Users experience the euphoria as a profound sense of control and well-being, as a satiation of need and relief from tension and frustration. Subjective time slows down.

Persian heroin is thought to come from Iran and other parts of the Near East where internal instability has created excellent conditions for the cultivation and transportation of narcotics. The distinctive characteristic of this type of heroin is its high level of purity and high quality. According to quantitative analysis, Persian heroin contains a high concentration of heroin (in some cases over 90%). Unlike street heroin, it can be rendered into a form suitable for snorting or smoking.

We at the Haight-Ashbury Free Medical Clinic began to see addiction to "rufus" in 1977. In 1978, clients of Iranian descent began to appear at our detoxification center for therapy. Their name for the drug was "dava," a Parsee word for "medicine." This is what they consider heroin to be within their own cultural context. Since 1980, use by white, middle-class abusers in the United States has been on the increase and spreading from major urban centers on both coasts to other parts of the country. Many abusers are among the affluent, upwardly mobile over-achievers in our professional world who use it in an "upper/downer" pattern along with cocaine freebasing.

Many addicts claim that the drug is too insoluble to "cook up" (dissolve into solution for injection) properly. Nevertheless, there has been a steady increase in the intravenous use of Persian. An acidic solution such as lemon juice is used to dissolve the heroin for injection. This form is often referred to as "lemon dope."

The most common means of abuse is by smoking or snorting. Smoking is either by direct combustion, alone or mixed with marijuana or tobacco, or by heating the powder and inhaling the vapor through a straw. This method, called "chasing the dragon," is also used with high-potency heroin in the Far East. Snorting (insufflation and absorption through the nasal mucous membrane) is the same method as is employed with cocaine, while "chasing the dragon" is somewhat similar to cocaine freebasing.

Dangers

With the purity of Persian heroin ranging as high as 92%, as compared with street heroin at 2 to 4%, there is a great danger of heroin overdose and death. The presence of high-quality heroin for sale has also prompted some dealers of street heroin to decrease the fillers in their product or to add such potent synthetic opioids as alpha methyl fentanyl. These efforts to enhance salability of street heroin increase the overdose hazard of these preparations. Conversely, additives such as instant coffee, used to make "white" look like Persian, increase the difficulty of diagnosis for overdose or addiction.

Persion heroin, like any form of heroin, can produce physical dependence (addiction) when used regularly. In general, daily use for 30 days is required for physical dependence to develop, but psychological dependence and narcotic hunger can develop in less time and with less frequent use.

The very fact that Persian heroin is smoked or snorted, rather than injected, leads many heroin abusers to the belief that they are not vulnerable to addiction. Clients are often surprised to discover that they are hooked without ever having stuck a needle into their arms. Physical addiction is a result of the drug itself, not of the route of administration. Some Persian users got started on the drug by using it to mediate the less desirable effects of cocaine freebasing and then develop a dependence to both drugs.

Emergency Treatment

The symptoms of heroin overdose are the combination of pinpointed pupils and declining level of consciousness. The level will decline all the way down to a comatose state. If untreated, it will often result in death. In the comatose state, the client's pupils may be dilated. An overdose can be reversed by the administration of naloxone, a narcotic antagonist that blocks opiate receptor sites until the heroin is metabolized and excreted. The patient should be kept under observation throughout this process so that the antagonist can be readministered if necessary.

Long-term Treatment

Withdrawal from heroin can be likened to a bad case of flu. There are no life-threatening qualities to heroin withdrawal, including high-potency

Persian heroin, and addicts may safely detoxify on their own. They may be more successful, however, and they will almost certainly be more comfortable if they place themselves in professional care. Withdrawal can be treated symptomatically, with nonnarcotic painkillers and medication for anxiety and diarrhea. There are a wide variety of methods of treating withdrawal, from "cold turkey" to acupuncture. Withdrawal symptoms of Persian heroin addicts treated at the Haight-Ashbury Free Medical Clinic are similar to those of other heroin addicts, but they are more severe and less responsive to treatment. The symptoms generally persist longer than those of addicts using ordinary street heroin. After successful detoxification, however, there is no higher rate of return to abuse than among other heroin clients.

MISCELLANEOUS NARCOTICS/ANALGESICS

At the start of this chapter we cited a number of substances that fall within the narcotic/analgesic category. We have explored the most notorious of these in depth in separate sections and have reviewed general narcotic treatment for abuse, addiction and overdose in the introduction. Here, we mention others, but to avoid repetition, we discuss only the points where they *differ* from other drugs in the general category. It should be kept in mind that treatment for overdoses and addiction is similar for all narcotics.

Alphaprodine (Nisentil®)

A piperidine derivative that has a rapid onset of analgesic effect but a short duration of action.

Anileridine (Levitine®)

Chemically related to meperidine but slightly more potent. Used for severe pain orally at 25 to 50 mg or intramuscularly at 40 mg.

Hydromorphone Hydrochloride (Dilaudid®)

Schedule II. Street names: First line, dillies. Used for moderate to severe pain due to surgery, cancer, trauma, colic, heart attack, or burns. This drug is chosen by many health professionals. Takes effect in about 15 to 30 minutes, peaks in 30 to 90 minutes, and lasts about 4 to 5 hours. Adult clinical dose is 2 mg every 4 to 6 hours.

Meperidine Hydrochloride (Demerol®, Pethadol®, etc.)

Schedule II. Street name: Cubes. Used for moderate to severe pain, severe migraine headaches, childbirth. Usually injected but may be given in pill form. Chemically incompatible with barbiturates. Takes effect in 10 to 15 minutes, peaks in 30 to 60 minutes and lasts 2 to 4 hours. Adult dosage is 50 to 150 mg every 3 to 4 hours.

Meperidine was originally introduced as an atropine-type antispasmodic. Its short duration and tissue irritation make it less desirable as a drug of abuse than other narcotics. On withdrawal, gastrointestinal problems may be lighter, but central nervous system problems are more pronounced than with other analgesics. Injection may be followed by severe hypotension, possibly caused by a histamine reaction. Abuse of this drug is high among health professionals who have relatively easy access to it.

Piminodine (Alvodine®), an analgesic, and diphenoxylate (Lomotil®), used for the control of diarrhea, are both closely related to meperidine.

In recent years, a meperidine analogue called MPPP that is manufactured in the drug underground has been found to cause a form of Parkinson's disease-like paralysis in abusers. This problem is discussed at length in the section on MPPP.

Nalbuphine Hydrochloride (Nubain®)

Chemically related to both the narcotic antagonist naloxone and the analgesic oxymorphone, nalbuphine is a potent analgesic with an onset of 2 to 3 minutes. It is used for the relief of moderate to severe pain, preoperative analgesia, as a supplement to surgical anesthesia, and obstetric analgesia during labor. Because it is partially a narcotic antagonist, it is thought to have a low abuse potential. However, abrupt withdrawal produces symptoms similar to those with any other narcotic.

Oxycodone Hydrochloride (Percocet®, Percodan®, Tylox®)

Schedule II. Used for mild to moderate pain, usually in combination with aspirin or acetaminophen. These additional ingredients may interfere with blood-clotting drugs.

Pentazocine (Talwin®)

Schedule IV. Talwin was developed in the course of narcotic antagonist research. It is injected subcutaneously or intramuscularly in 20 to 40 mg doses for analgesia. Alone it is thought to have a low dependence potential because of a flattening response curve; that is, higher doses do not increase the potency. However, it was a component in T's and Blues

(Talwin® and tripelennamine) used in the midwest as a substitute for heroin (and dealt with in the section on drug combinations). Talwin® now comes in combination with the narcotic antagonist naloxone to discourage this abuse.

Propoxyphene Hydrochloride (Darvon®)

Although usually used for mild analgesia, Darvon® is considered a narcotic analgesic by international accord. It tends to be effective as a symptomatic medication for narcotic withdrawal, but this indication has been blocked by United States adherence to international accord.

Butorphanol Tartrate (Stadol®)

Listed as a sterile, parenteral, narcotic antagonist/agonist, analgesic. Chemical name: levo-N-cyclobutylmethyl-6, 10ab-dihydroxy-1,2,3, 9,10, 10a-hexahydro-(4H)-10, 4a-iminoethanophen-nanthreme tartrate. White crystalline substance soluble in aqueous solution. A potent analgesic comparable to morphine with an effect of 3 to 4 hours. Used for relief of moderate to severe pain. Because of its antagonist properties, its use is not recommended for persons who are physically dependent on narcotics.

Central Nervous System Depressants

HISTORICAL PERSPECTIVE

The central nervous system depressants form a large category of drugs that are often divided into overlapping groups: sedatives, hypnotics, sedative-hypnotics, minor and major tranquilizers, and so on. As we have found with narcotic/analgesics, the use of at least one CNS depressant goes far back into prehistory. For the CNS depressant group, that representative drug is alcohol.

Alcohol occurs naturally through certain chemobiological processes and was doubtless discovered rather than synthesized. This discovery probably took place when one of our well-removed cave-dwelling ancestors got tipsy on fermented fruit and grunted this experience to pretribal neighbors. Since that antedeluvian time, alcohol has become so much a part of human culture that we often forget that it is a drug. Except for certain religious groups, and some U.S. citizens during Prohibition (1919 to 1933) most people regard alcohol as an acceptable recreational drug. In a sense, it is a dangerous psychoactive substance that we have given ourselves permission to use in a nonmedical way. Sidney Cohen, MD, pointed out in his book *The Substance Abuse Problems* (Cohen, 1981) that "if alcohol were a newly discovered drug, and if it were submitted to the F.D.A. for marketing, it could hardly be approved for sale. The adverse effects and complications of extensive use are simply too many."

In many definitions of the overall group, narcotics and analgesics are included within the broad framework of central nervous system depressants. We have separated them out for a variety of reasons, including pharmacologic action and differences in the ways these drugs are abused, create dependency, and are treated. One major difference is that withdrawal from narcotic analgesics is uncomfortable but is not a threat to health or life. Withdrawal from other depressant drugs can be life threatening.

There are, however, many similarities between the two groups. Historically, they have often been used to treat similar problems. Both drug groups have a "downer" effect when compared with the "upper" effect of stimulants. Nevertheless, the sedative-hypnotics have fulfilled medical needs quite apart from those served by the narcotic analgesics.

Although they may seem to be by-products of our current hypertechno-
logical society, anxiety and insomnia have been part of the human condition for a long time. The treatment of these conditions, of convulsions,
and of certain forms of epilepsy form the most common indications for
sedative-hypnotic drugs.

In the 19th century, these afflictions were treated with opiates, bromide
salts, chloral hydrate (developed in 1869), paraldehyde (developed in
1882), and alcohol. Each of these substances had its problems as a depressant. The bromides could cause chronic bromide poisoning, and
many patients refused to take alcohol, while chloral hydrate and paraldehyde had objectionable taste and smell. As a consequence, the development of barbiturates was hailed as a major breakthrough.

The sedative-hypnotic barbiturates are all derived from barbituric acid.
First obtained from uric acid, barbituric acid was synthesized in Germany
by Dr. Adolf van Baeyer in 1864. Conrad and Guthzeit synthesized the
first barbiturate, 5,5-diethylbarbituric acid (barbital) in 1882. In 1903,
Emile Fischer and Baron Josef von Mering introduced barbital into clinical medicine under the trade name Veronal®. Phenobarbital, which has
remained the "Model T" of sedative-hypnotics, first appeared on the
market in 1912 as Luminal®. Intoxication with barbiturates is qualitatively similar to intoxication with alcohol, and similar problems of abuse
became apparent through the 1920s, 1930s, and 1940s as the abuse of
these drugs escalated.

The history of sedative-hypnotic drugs has been a history of attempts
to find a drug or family of drugs that produces the desired effects without
the risk of dependence and debilitating or life-threatening side effects and
overdoses. Time and again, a new drug in this class has been developed
and touted as "safe and effective." The drug has achieved high status
within the pharmacopeia, only to fall as reports of abuse, overdose, and
death overtake it. Perhaps we need to consider the possibility that any
chemical substance that effectively makes us feel good and curbs anxiety,
depression, and insomnia is going to create dependence and abuse in
certain people. Perhaps someday we will develop mature ways of dealing
with the drugs we have and our reaction to them, instead of inventing new
ones that merely start the whole tragic cycle rolling again.

Under pressure to find a "safe" substitute for barbiturates, which had
been developed as a "safe" substitute for bromides, the pharmaceutical
industry devised glutethimide, ethchlorvynol and methyprylon. These
drugs appeared on the market as nonbarbiturate sedative-hypnotics in
1954 and 1955, but they were found to have the same potential for abuse
as the barbiturates they were meant to replace.

A prime example of the rise and fall of a sedative-hypnotic can be seen
in the history of methaqualone. Sold in the United States as Quaalude®

and overseas as Mandrax®, methaqualone was a synthetic organic chemical unrelated structurally to the barbiturates. Originally developed to fight malaria, it was remarketed as a sedative after its sedative effects became apparent. Sold as a safe, effective, and nonaddicting substitute for barbiturates, it rapidly became America's sixth best-selling sedative. It did even better as a street recreational drug after picking up an undeserved reputation as an aphrodisiac. Within 15 years of its introduction, methaqualone had become number three on the government's list of most-abused drugs. In 1984, the sole manufacturer of this drug in the United States ceased production.

Major tranquilizers like the phenothiazines, which include chlorpromazine (Thorazine®), are not usually subject to recreational abuse. Problems with these drugs most often entail misprescription and lack of understanding of their effects by health professionals. They are not considered to be addictive, and although a few deaths have been attributed to the ingestion of high doses, it is difficult to use them to commit suicide. These drugs have come under recent media attention because of their development of extrapyramidal symptoms that include facial and other abnormal movements of the head and neck, as well as such parkinson syndrome-like symptoms as tremor at rest, rigidity, and shuffling walk.

A final group of central nervous system depressants that has gained wide acceptance and use in the medical community is the benzodiazepines. These drugs are also called the minor tranquilizers. They have been developed over the past 20 years, starting with chlordiazepoxide (Librium®), which was quickly followed by diazepam (Valium®). Since then, a variety of benzodiazepines have been synthesized. These may range in duration of effects and specific indications, but they are all crosstolerant and chemically similar.

Safer than the barbiturates and other sedative-hypnotics, the benzodiazepines now form the backbone for treatment. Valium® has received notoriety as a dependence producer, but it remains the second most-prescribed medication in the United States. For a long time, it was thought that the physical dependence-producing dose of any of the benzodiazepines was at least five times greater than the usually prescribed therapeutic dose. Recent studies have shown, however, that people who are vulnerable to addictive disease, as evidenced by a family history of drug addiction or alcoholism, do develop dependence to these drugs and exhibit symptoms when withdrawn from therapeutic dosage levels. It therefore behooves physicians to monitor any long-term benzodiazepine prescribees for possible dependence, and to take appropriate steps if dependence does appear. No physician should, however, abruptly terminate a course of any sedative-hypnotic medication with a possibly dependent patient. Such a move could well prove life threatening.

In the main, benzodiazepines have a favorable therapeutic ratio with well-established therapeutic indications, relatively few side effects, and less overdose potential than most sedative-hypnotic drugs.

Sedative-hypnotic drugs are all cross tolerant and can produce a life-threatening effect when mixed or used concurrently. This effect is caused by the buildup of one while the other continues in the system at full strength. While alcohol is being digested, for example, successive doses of barbiturates may be building in strength in the brain toward a potentially fatal overdose.

ACUTE SEDATIVE-HYPNOTIC TOXICITY

Intoxication with all sedative-hypnotic drugs is similar and resembles symptoms produced by that most familiar of intoxicants, alcohol. The exact effects of this intoxication may vary from time to time, even with the same individual. In recreational abuse, the desired effect is generally one of "disinhibition euphoria," a state in which mood is elevated; self-criticism, anxiety, and guilt are reduced; and the user feels an increase in energy and self-confidence. Although euphoria may occur with sedative-hypnotics, the mood may be quite labile and the individual may also experience sadness, rapidly fluctuating mood shifts, irritability, hypochondriacal concerns, increased anxiety, and agitation. It is the euphoria of short-acting barbiturates and certain other sedative-hypnotics that makes them appealing as intoxicants, but this state of disinhibition euphoria is not necessarily synonymous with intoxication.

Intoxicated individuals commonly show unsteady gait, slurred speech, sustained vertical and horizontal nystagmus (eye wiggle), and poor judgment. Their subjective state is often unpleasant or dysphoric. Regardless of the mood effects, sedative-hypnotic intoxication produces a reduction in the ability to make accurate judgments and markedly impairs motor coordination. Barbiturates are well absorbed from the stomach, but the short-acting ones absorb more readily than the longer-acting ones. Alcohol enhances absorption and produces an additive sedative-hypnotic effect.

The sodium salts of barbiturates can be injected intramuscularly or intravenously, although the solutions, including those prepared by pharmaceutical companies specifically for injection, are very alkaline. The needle sites seem especially prone to irritation and abscess. In some cases where users have indulged in frequent subcutaneous injection, the needle abscesses have been notably disfiguring.

The greatest danger with acute sedative-hypnotic toxicity is an actual overdose. Overdosage may result from one drug or from the additive effect of several substances. Most often another sedative hypnotic is taken concurrently with alcohol.

TREATMENT OF A SEDATIVE-HYPNOTIC OVERDOSE

Overdose patients can be awake, semicomatose, or comatose depending on the degree of CNS depression. There are specific procedures for each of these states.

Awake Patient

Respiration, blood pressure, and pulse rate are evaluated, the patient's pupils are checked, a heart and lung examination is performed, and bowel sounds are evaluated. Pertinent information is obtained from the patient, if possible, or from the persons who brought the patient in, to determine what intoxicants have been ingested. Unfortunately, even when a friend accompanies a patient, the drug history obtained may be unreliable. Therefore, if feasible, the material the patient has ingested should be subjected to toxicologic analysis as quickly as possible. If the patient is awake after the history and physical workup are completed, vomiting should be induced with syrup of ipecac rather than using lavage. Lavage with a large tube is extremely difficult when the patient is semicomatose or awake. Furthermore, it is important to induce vomiting, not only to eliminate any psychoactive drug still remaining in the stomach, but to obtain a toxicological analysis of the stomach's contents.

Vomiting is also preferable to lavage in an awake patient because the first part of the small bowel is also emptied by vomiting, whereas gastric lavage clears only the stomach contents. After vomiting has been induced, the patients' vital signs and mental status should be checked every 15 minutes to determine whether they are becoming stuporous or comatose. If, after a few hours, it is apparent that the CNS depression is not progressing, the patient can be released to appropriate medical, detoxification, or psychiatric aftercare facilities.

Semicomatose Patient

If the patient is semicomatose, an endotracheal tube cannot be inserted to protect the airway. Vomiting should not be induced because semicomatose patients are likely to aspirate the stomach's contents. With the patient in a semirecumbent position, careful gastric lavage with 10 to 15 liters of lavage fluid is indicated if it can be determined that the drug was ingested within 4 hours of treatment. A slurry of activated charcoal can be instilled into the stomach through the lavage tube and left in the stomach to retard the absorption of any material that is not removed by lavage.

The advantage of removing the unabsorbed drug from the stomach must be weighed against the danger of pulmonary aspiration that may occur during lavage. Some physicians believe that in a medical setting where prompt treatment of respiratory insufficiency can be instituted, the danger of lavage with attendant risk of aspiration is greater than the danger of progressive respiratory insufficiency. Therefore, they do not lavage unless the patient can tolerate an endotracheal tube.

An evaluation of arterial blood gases can be used to determine the degree of respiratory insufficiency. The patient's EKG and respiration should be monitored continuously until the patient regains consciousness and is mentally alert. He or she should then be released to appropriate medical, detoxification, or psychiatric aftercare facilities.

Comatose Patient

When the patient comes into the emergency room or treatment center after ingesting sedative-hypnotics and is comatose, a life-threatening emergency is present and the following steps should be taken as quickly as possible:

1. Clear the airway.
2. Establish an intravenous fluid system to maintain the cardiovascular system, and administer drugs rapidly.
3. Obtain a brief history and physical examination.
4. Take the vital signs.
5. Insert an endotracheal tube to guard the airway.
6. Perform gastric lavage with fluid containing activated charcoal to remove any remaining psychoactive drug from the stomach and obtain material for toxicologic analysis.

After all of the above procedures have been completed, arterial blood should be drawn and analyzed for blood gases to evaluate the degree of respiratory sufficiency. Two major prognostic signs of approaching respiratory failure and cardiovascular collapse are respiratory acidosis (the result of depressed ventilation with retained CO_2) and low blood pressure. After patients have received emergency treatment, they should be transferred to the intensive care unit, which will continue to provide the following: respirator-assisted ventilation, intravenous fluids, cardiovascular monitoring, careful monitoring of urinary output, and intensive nursing care.

After emergency treatment of the comatose patient has been completed, some physicians initiate measures to increase the excretion of barbiturates or other sedative-hypnotics through forced diuresis, hemodialysis, or peritoneal dialysis. Alkalinization of the urine can be used to increase excretion of phenobarbital. These procedures, however, are not without risk and have their own rate of morbidity.

The most common cause of sedative hypnotic overdose is a suicide attempt. This is followed by cases of additive effect, usually mixing a medical sedative-hypnotic with alcohol. An added danger with these drugs is such chronic morbidity as tissue necrosis and brain damage. These may produce long-term disability.

CHRONIC SEDATIVE-HYPNOTIC TOXICITY

Sedative-hypnotics can produce psychological dependence, physical dependence, and tolerance. Psychological dependence refers to a strong need to experience the drug effects repeatedly, even in the absence of physical dependence. Physical dependence refers to the establishment of objective signs of withdrawal which occur after the drug is abruptly stopped, and tolerance refers to the adaption of the body to the drug in such a manner that larger doses are required to produce the original effects. With sedative-hypnotics, two types of tolerance may develop. Drug-disposition tolerance develops from activation of drug-metabolizing enzyme systems in the liver capable of destroying barbiturates and other sedative-hypnotics more rapidly. Pharmacodynamic tolerance is due to the adaptation of the central nervous system to the presence of the drug. As the individual increases the dose to maintain the same level of intoxication, the margin between the intoxicating dose and the lethal dose becomes smaller.

Some people are prone to overuse any drug that will lessen their worries or anxieties. The intent of their drug usage is to maintain an anxiety-free state. These are usually people who do not identify with any drug-using population. They tend to be middle class or blue collar and 30 to 50 years old or older. The drug was probably prescribed by a physician.

They find that sedative-hypnotics make coping with life easier, and as tolerance to the tranquilizing and sedative effects develops, they increase their dose — often without their physician's knowledge. They may see several physicians, in fact, none of whom may be aware that the patient is abusing the drugs they are prescribing. The abuse pattern of these patients may go unidentified for some time until confusion, irritability, decreased ability to work, and episodes of acute intoxication with slurred speech and staggering gait finally draw attention to it.

Recreational abuse of sedative-hypnotics is usually seen in a younger or poorer population. Use may be episodic. High doses may be taken orally, or capsules may be dissolved in water and injected primarily for the "rush," a drowsy warm feeling experienced immediately after injection. Barbiturates and other sedative drugs may be used as part of an "upper/downer" pattern to mediate the less desirable effects of chronic stimulant use. Heroin addicts may supplement their drug with sedative-hypnotics when their supply of heroin is low — or opiates may be cut with barbiturates.

DETOXIFICATION FROM SEDATIVE-HYPNOTICS

The symptoms of sedative-hypnotic withdrawal do not follow a specific sequence but can include anxiety, tremors, nightmares, insomnia, anorexia, nausea, vomiting, postural hypotension, seizures, delirium, and hyperpyrexia (fever). The syndrome is similar for all sedative-hypnotics. The time course, however, depends on the particular drug involved. With pentobarbital, secobarbital, meprobamate, and methaqualone, withdrawal symptoms may begin 12 to 24 hours after the last dose and may peak in intensity between 24 and 72 hours. The withdrawal reactions to phenobarbital, diazepam, and chlordiazepoxide develop more slowly and peak on the fifth to eighth day.

During the first 1 to 5 days of untreated sedative-hypnotic withdrawal, the EEG may show a paroxysmal burst of high-voltage, slow-frequency activity which precedes the development of seizures. The withdrawal delirium may include disorientation to time, place, and situation, as well as visual and auditory hallucinations. The delirium generally follows a period of insomnia. Some individuals may have only delirium, others only seizures, and some may have both delirium and convulsion.

There are two major methods of detoxifying the sedative-hypnotic dependent patient: (1) gradual withdrawal of the addicting agent and (2) the substitution of long-acting phenobarbital for the addicting agent while gradually withdrawing the substitute drug. Either method makes use of the stepwise withdrawal and avoids the dangerous and often life-threatening abrupt withdrawal. We prefer the phenobarbital substitution in that it permits a withdrawal characterized by fewer fluctuations in blood levels of the drug throughout the day and thus enables the safe use of smaller doses. Lethal doses are several times greater than toxic doses and the signs of toxicity are easy to observe. Also, phenobarbital does not produce the behavioral problems commonly associated with disinhibition euphoria.

The phenobarbital withdrawal equivalents vary, but Table 1 gives daily dosages equivalent to 30 mg of phenobarbital for withdrawal management:

Table 1. Daily Dosages Equivalent to 30 mg Phenobarbital

Amobarbital	100
Butabarbital	60
Pentobarbital	100

Secobarbital	100
Chloral hydrate	500
Ethchlorvynol (Placidyl®)	350
Glutethimide (Doriden®)	250
Meprobamate (Equanil®, Miltown®)	400
Methaqualone (Quaalude®)	300
Methyprylon (Noludar®)	100
Chlordiazepoxide (Librium®)	100
Clorazepate (Tranxene®)	50
Diazepam (Valium®)	50
Flurazepam (Dalmane®)	30
Oxazepam (Serax®)	100

On the basis of the phenobarbital dosage calculated using the withdrawal equivalence, the patient is maintained on the oral dose schedule for 2 days and then withdrawn with a graded reduction not to exceed 30 mg per day. Regardless of the calculated dosage, doses of phenobarbital should not exceed 500 mg per day.

If the patient is in acute withdrawal and in danger of having seizures, one may administer the initial dose of phenobarbital by injection. We recommend 200 mg intramuscularly for stabilization. If nystagmus and other signs of intoxication develop following the intramuscular dosage, it is doubtful that the individual is dependent.

If the patient is dependent on alcohol as well as another sedative-hypnotic, as is often the case, the phenobarbital equivalence of the alcohol is added to the phenobarbital equivalence for the other sedative-hypnotic in determining the total daily dosage. The alcohol withdrawal equivalents are:

Average daily quantity of alcohol consumed for more than 1 month	Equivalent in phenobarbital
1 ounce of 80-proof alcohol	15 mg
1 pint	240 mg
1 fifth (4/5 quart)	380 mg
1 quart	480 mg

If the patient has grossly overstated the magnitude of the addiction, toxic symptoms will occur during the first day or so of treatment. The problem can be managed by omitting one or more doses of phenobarbital and recalculating the daily dose (Smith, 1984; Seymour et al., 1982).

ALCOHOL

Category: Use and purchasing of recreational products containing alcohol is regulated by state governments. There is currently a move to make age 21 the nationwide lower limit for purchasing alcoholic beverages.

Chemical names: Ethanol or ethyl alcohol

Product names: Gin, vodka, bourbon, scotch, rye, whiskey, brandy, wine, beer, fortified wine

Street names: Hootch, booze, moonshine, white lightning, ol' red eye, poison, juice, hair of the dog, cocktails

Description: Pure ethyl alcohol is a highly volatile colorless liquid. Alcohol is most often found in a variety of natural juices and fruit and vegetable mashes as a product of fermentation. In this process, yeast and other microorganisms break down the sugar in the vegetable matter into alcohol. Potency can be increased through either fortification, the adding of additional alcohol, or distillation, vaporization and condensation of the product to produce a more concentrated form.

Wine, beer, pulque, and fermented yak's milk are some of the intoxicants that are the direct product of fermentation. Port, sherry, Madeira, and Malaga are types of fortified wines. Brandy, liquors, whiskeys, gins, and vodkas are examples of even more potent distilled beverages.

Means of ingestion: Alcohol preparations are usually imbibed in liquid form either by themselves (straight) or diluted with other liquids. There is a vast pharmacopeia of alcohol preparations for recreational use. Alcohol also serves as the medium for a number of medicines. Most medicines referred to as "tinctures" or "elixirs" are dissolved in alcohol. Alcoholic beverages are also used as a flavoring in cooking, but in most recipes the alcohol content is boiled away, leaving only a residual taste in the food. So far as we know, no studies have been done on the psychoactive effect of alcohol vapor on cooks.

General Information

Alcohol is so much a part of Western civilization that we tend to forget that it is a drug. It is, indeed, our oldest psychoactive drug. With the exception of certain religious groups, such as Near Eastern Muslim and some Christian fundamentalist sects, alcohol is ingested in some form or other by most peoples of the world. In our own culture, it is used both as a social lubricant and as a religious ceremonial ingredient, although its religious use consists more often of a symbolic sip than a means to holy intoxication.

In classical Greece and Rome, wine itself was considered holy and was represented by its own gods, Dionysus and Bacchus respectively. These ancients diluted their wine with water, considering it far too intoxicating to be taken straight. They also mixed their wine with herbs at religious ceremonies, giving rise to speculation that these rites made use of additional psychoactive substances with their alcohol. To the north, tribes favored beer made from grains and a fermented honey called mead. Distilled spirits were a recent addition, having been developed by alchemists in the late Middle Ages.

Alcohol is produced by the digestion of the sugar in vegetable matter by a variety of yeasts and other microorganisms. This process is called fermentation. If fruits, especially grapes, are used, the product is called wine. If grains are used, it is beer. There are also a wide variety of regional intoxicants produced by fermentation, such as pulque (made from the maguey cactus) in Mexico and Central America, and fermented yak butter in Central Asia as well as sake, the rice wine of Japan. Alcohol has a low vaporizing point and can be distilled into high-potency products such as brandies, whiskeys, and cordials. The forms and mixtures in which alcohol is used are legion, as are the myths connected with this drug.

In most cultures, including our own, alcohol can be used in moderation for relaxation and euphoria and as a social lubricant. In the United States it was briefly outlawed by constitutional amendment, but enforcement of that ban proved impossible. Today, alcohol is one of the few recreational drugs sanctioned for use by adults. Its production is a major industry, complete with a wide variety of retail outlets for its sale and consumption.

Alcohol has many industrial uses, including combustion with gasoline as gasohol. Although it is a medium for many medicines, it has only one medical indication of its own. That is for treatment of methanol poisoning (Becker et al., 1974). It is used externally as a disinfectant.

Dangers

Ten million people in the United States are dependent on alcohol. Ninety percent of all assaults, 50 to 60% of all murders, over half the rapes and sexual attacks on children, and from one-third to half of all arrests involve intoxication by alcohol. The suicide rate among alcoholics is 6 to 20 times higher than in the general population. Hundreds of thousands of divorces, desertions, and separations involve alcohol. Industry loses five billion dollars a year and the government another half billion through the effects of alcohol on employees. Although about 90% of alcohol users may suffer few ill effects from moderate use, alcohol obviously has its dark side.

Chronic alcoholism causes damage to the brain, nervous system, liver, and pancreas that in time may be irreversible — in fact, these represent the only drug sequelae that have been clinically proved to be irreversible.

Alcohol produces tension, depression, and other symptoms that account for a fifth to a quarter of all psychiatric hospital admissions. Alcohol intoxication may cause loss of judgment, foolhardy behavior, industrial and automobile accidents, blackouts, loss of memory, cardiac arrest, and death. Withdrawal from incidental intoxication may cause headaches, nausea, loss of appetite, shakiness, and muddled thinking. Withdrawal from heavy, long-term intoxication may cause grand mal convulsions, toxic psychosis with hallucinations, tremulousness, agitation, and death.

There is a high propensity for alcohol addiction, or alcoholism, marked by the addictive disease symptoms of compulsion, loss of control, and continued use despite adverse consequences. We do not know if this propensity is hereditary, but statistics indicate that a child with one alcoholic parent is 30 times more likely to become an alcoholic than one with no family history of alcoholism or drug abuse. That differential rises to 400 times if both parents are alcoholics or addicts (Smith, 1985).

Alcoholics cannot control their intake: One drink is too many and a thousand are not enough. Incidental intoxication can be life threatening, both physiologically through sedative-hypnotic cardiovascular suppression and physically, through alcohol-induced violence and accidents. Over 50% of fatal traffic accidents involve alcohol. In recent years, such organizations as Mothers Against Drunk Driving (MADD) have forced recognition of this fact and are helping create major revisions in state and national drunk driving laws and prosecution.

Chronic intoxication along with poor diet can cause cirrhosis of the liver, peripheral neuritis, and a host of other degenerative diseases, while withdrawal can precipitate potentially fatal seizures, psychoses and the DTs, or delirium tremens (disorientation of time, place, and person coupled with continuous hallucinations that the client does not recognise as hallucinations).

Alcohol use by pregnant women can result in a variety of birth defects known collectively as fetal alcohol syndrome (FAS). Alcohol has a dangerous additive effect when used with marijuana, or any sedative-hypnotics (of which it is one) including barbiturates, methaqualone, or benzodiazepines (Librium®, Valium®, etc.). It also can be a secondary addictive component when used to counter the effects of cocaine and amphetamines.

If alcohol were a new drug being reviewed by the U.S. Food and Drug

Administration, it would never be approved for use (Cohen, 1981).

Emergency Treatment

Time is the best healer for incidental intoxication and withdrawal, i.e., being drunk and hung over. Never try to sober someone up with coffee; all you get is a wide-awake drunk. In the hung-over state, liquids can hasten recovery and moderate exercise such as walking in the fresh air can help. Use of alcohol to nullify the effects of a hangover (the "hair of the dog" idea) is a step toward addiction. In extreme situations, the intoxicated individual should be taken to an emergency room or poison center for treatment and observation.

Long-term Treatment

Alcoholic detoxification should be undertaken in an inpatient setting and is similar to any sedative-hypnotic detoxification. Withdrawal can involve a variety of symptoms, some of which can be life threatening, so the patient needs to be under observation. We use phenobarbital substitution and step-down procedures as outlined in the section on sedative-hypnotic treatment.

Chronic intoxication and compulsive drinking should be dealt with through long-term therapy and support. Alcoholics Anonymous and other recovery-oriented programs are recommended. Recovery orientation is based on the adoption of a way of life that is rewarding without the use of alcohol or any other psychoactive drugs. Because of the propensity toward alcoholism in children of alcoholics, these children should be advised of the risk and counseled in a nonjudgmental, nonmoralistic manner.

AMYL, BUTYL, AND ISOBUTYL NITRITE

Category: Amyl nitrite crushable inhalers available by prescription. Other forms on open sale as "room odorizers."

Product names: Amyl nitrite inhalers, Locker Room, Rush, Heart On

Street names: Nitrites, poppers, snappers, bananas, rush, liquid incense

Description: Amyl nitrite crushable inhalers are small glass vials covered with a cloth web to keep glass fragments from extruding when the vapor is released. Other preparations come in spray cans.

Means of ingestion: Inhalation.

General Information

The alkyl nitrites are aliphatic esters of nitrous acid. Although these esters include numerous others that have similar effects and abuse potential, the most frequently used as intoxicants are amyl, butyl, and isobutyl nitrite (Nickerson et al., 1979). Amyl nitrite was originally available without a prescription at drugstores. It was packaged in crushable containers popularly known as "poppers." These poppers are used medically to relieve angina pectoris (heart-related chest pains) and for the treatment of cyanide poisoning. In angina, the nitrites work by dilating blood vessels near the heart so that more blood can reach it. Nitroglycerin — ordinarily not an intoxicant — is also used for this purpose. In the treatment of cyanide poisoning, amyl nitrite changes the hemoglobin in blood to methemoglobin, which combines with cyanide and keeps it from doing cellular damage within the body (Inaba, 1974a).

The primary effect of these drugs is the relaxation of all smooth muscles in the body, including smooth muscle in blood vessels. This relaxation may allow a greater flow of oxygenated blood to the brain or may decrease the flow. The effects of inhalation last about 30 seconds: Blood pressure reaches its lowest point in 30 seconds and returns to normal at about 90 seconds. On inhalation, there is a distinct "rush" similar to that experienced on inhaling nitrous oxide — a related substance used as an anesthetic. This rush may be followed by severe headaches, but tolerance to this unpleasant side effect increases rapidly with use of the drug. The relaxation of blood vessels can cause a distinct flushing of the neck and face. Some swelling is possible as well.

The recreational popularity of the alkyl nitrites results from their reputation as aphrodisiacs (substances that in some way improve sexual performance or enjoyment). To gain this effect, the nitrites are usually inhaled just before sexual orgasm. The reported intensification and prolongation of orgasm may be an illusion, however. The rush, involving dizziness and giddiness, may cause a reduction of social and sexual inhibitions along with a time distortion. This combination may lead to a sense of prolonged orgasm in both men and women.

On the other hand, increased flow of blood to sexual organs may well increase sensitivity to sexual activity. Some homosexual men have reported that the collateral relaxation of the anal sphincter (made of smooth-muscle tissue) facilitates certain forms of sexual activity (Latimer, 1981).

After many complaints that these drugs were being abused, the Food and Drug Administration returned amyl nitrite inhalers to prescription status in 1969. Since that time, sales of nitrite based "room odorizers" with such names as "Locker Room," "Rush," and "Heart On" have increased dramatically. Butyl nitrite and isobutyl nitrite have identical pharmaceutical effects to amyl nitrite.

Dangers

Tolerance to the physiological effects of the nitrites occurs rapidly and can be pronounced within a few weeks. This tolerance is lost within a few days after suspending use, leaving the user vulnerable again to severe headaches following resumed use.

Excessive use may result in nitrite poisoning or excessive methemoglobinemia. Symptoms of this may include severe vomiting, cyanosis (blue-tinged lips and skin), shock, or unconsciousness. Blood vessel dilation may bring about a sudden drop in blood pressure and loss of consciousness (orthostatic hypotension), especially if one gets up quickly after inhaling the drug. An increase in heart rate and palpitations makes nitrites risky for anyone with heart problems. Breathing any inhalant over a prolonged period and with restricted or nonexistent ventilation can cause oxygen deprivation, asphyxiation, and possibly death (Inaba, 1974b). There have been isolated reports of persons sustaining myocardial infarctions (heart attacks) after the blood pressure drop associated with nitrite inhalation, but no fatalities have been recorded.

The Centers for Disease Control in Atlanta are investigating the possibility that inhalant nitrites (along with many other elements in the gay lifestyle) may in some way contribute to the development of acquired immune deficiency syndrome (AIDS), but at this time there is no scientific indication whatsoever of any such relationship.

A statistical link has long been established between nitrite compounds in general and the development of certain forms of cancer, but its relevance to occasional nitrite inhalers is unknown. This nitrite/cancer link is most commonly associated with regular ingestion of food preservatives and other chemical additives.

Emergency Treatment

The headaches that result from nitrite inhalation are short-lived and disappear with abstinence.

Overdose on the nitrites requires that adequate respiration and cardiac blood flow be maintained. Occasionally, cardiopulmonary resuscitation (CPR) is required. If a person passes out from the sudden blood pressure drop, standard hypotensive therapy—such as simply elevating the feet higher than the head to promote a return of blood to the brain—will ordinarily suffice.

Long-term Treatment

Compulsive use of nitrite inhalation should be approached with education and counseling. A recovery model including abstinence is most effective.

BARBITURATES

Chemical names: 5,5-diethylbarbituric acid, etc.

Category: Different products are in different schedules. For example, Seconal®, Amytal®, and Nembutal® are all Schedule II, Butisol® is Schedule III, and Luminal® is Schedule IV.

Product names: Thiopental (Pentothal®), amobarbital (Amytal®), pentobarbital (Nembutal®), secobarbital (Seconal®), Butabarbital (Butisol®), phenobarbital (Luminal®), etc.

Street names: Barbs, downers, yellow jackets, reds

Description: Barbiturates comprise a wide variety of tablets and capsules as well as injectable forms.

Means of ingestion: Either swallowed in pill or capsule form or injected.

General Information

Barbiturates are a group of sedative-hypnotic drugs that are derived from barbituric acid. This substance was synthesized in Germany by Dr. Adolf von Baeyer in 1864. Conrad and Guthzeit synthesized 5,5-diethylbarbituric acid (barbital) in 1882, and in 1903 Emile Fischer and Baron Josef von Mering introduced barbital into clinical medicine under the trade name Veronal (Smith et al., 1979).

The family of drugs that descended from barbital have replaced the earlier bromides as the "backbone" sedative-hypnotics used in medical treatment. They are used for a number of treatment indications. In the following list, we have classified them in order by duration of effects and have indicated the principal use and generic/trade names:

- *Ultrashort acting* (1/4 to 3 hours): Anesthetic induction (thiopental/ Pentothal®)
- *Short-acting* (3 to 6 hours): Hypnotic, preoperative sedation, injected for rapid seizure control (amobarbital/Amytal; pentobarbital/ Nembutal; secobarbital/Seconal)
- *Intermediate-acting* (6 to 12 hours): Daytime sedation (butabarbital/ Butisol®)
- *Long-acting* (12 to 24 hours): Control of epilepsy, daytime sedation, treatment of sedative-hypnotic withdrawal (phenobarbital/Luminal®) (Wesson & Smith, 1977)

Intoxication with barbiturates is qualitatively similar to intoxication with alcohol. The effect most users are seeking is "disinhibition euphoria" involving an elevation of mood and a reduction of self-critical introspection, anxiety, and guilt.

There was a major outbreak of high-dose intravenous barbiturate abuse in the drug subculture of the late 1960s. In the 1970s, these drugs had a prominent role in what came to be recognized as "middle-class polydrug abuse." Although barbiturates are the second most commonly prescribed drug group in the United States, the recreational use of these drugs has decreased in recent years, and other sedative-hypnotics with fewer undesirable side effects (or seemingly fewer) have come into favor. Barbiturates are often used in conjunction with stimulants in an upper/downer abuse pattern. They may also be used to supplement heroin when that drug is weak or scarce (Smith & Wesson, 1973).

Dangers

Barbiturate intoxication reduces one's ability to make accurate judgments and greatly impairs motor coordination. Although barbiturates may produce euphoria, the user might instead experience sadness, rapidly fluctuating mood shifts, irritability, hypochondria, increased anxiety, and agitation. Feelings of aggression, paranoia and anger may be acted out inappropriately as acts of violence. Intoxicated individuals commonly show unsteady gait, slurred speech, jerky eye movement (nystagmus), and poor judgment (Irwin, 1984).

Because the gap between an intoxicating dose and a fatal dose is small and can be made smaller by sedative-hypnotic tolerance, a sedative-hypnotic overdose is a life-threatening emergency. The signs and symptoms of barbiturate overdoses must be interpreted quickly and accurately and acted upon appropriately. These signs and symptoms include those listed above for intoxication and go on to include slowed reactions, lethargy, and progressive respiratory depression characterized by shallow, irregular breathing. Overdose can lead to coma and death (Smith & Wesson, 1974).

The danger of overdose is especially acute with barbiturates because, with prolonged use, the effective dosage level keeps rising while the overdose level remains relatively constant. Also, alcohol and other sedative hypnotics, including methaqualone and the benzodiazepines (Valium®, Librium®, Ativan®, etc.), have an additive effect when mixed with barbiturates, making the mixture potentially more deadly than each drug would be on its own.

Solutions of barbiturates irritate body tissues, and cellulitis can result from injection of these drugs as well as multiple needle abscesses. Accidental injection into an artery can cause severe blood vessel constriction and reduction of blood and oxygen supplies to the extremities, causing gangrene and in some cases necessitating amputation.

Like all sedative-hypnotics, barbiturates can produce tolerance, psychological dependence, and physical dependence. Withdrawal symptoms may include anxiety, tremors, sleeplessness, loss of appetite and weight (anorexia), nausea, vomiting, dizziness, and abdominal cramps. Several days after withdrawal begins, the user may experience delirium, delusions, and hallucinations, although the worst period of withdrawal is usually the second to fourth days after last use. Throughout withdrawal, there is a danger of grand mal seizures that may be fatal.

Emergency Treatment

A barbiturate overdose is a life-threatening emergency. It cannot be reversed with stimulants. If the patient is awake, try to keep him or her awake and moving. Otherwise, keep the patient warm and elevate the feet until the patient can be moved to an emergency treatment facility for definitive treatment. Fast action can save lives.

When the patient arrives at an emergency room, the condition should be rapidly assessed. If the patient is awake, vomiting should be induced and samples of the vomitus, blood, and urine and (if possible) the drug, should be taken for toxicologic analysis. If the patient is semiconscious and cannot tolerate an endotracheal tube, the airway should be cleared, vomiting should not be induced, and gastric lavage should be started. Cardiovascular and respiratory status should be monitored and an intravenous catheter inserted.

Whether or not the patient is conscious, emergency-room observation should be continued if the patient's condition becomes stable. Emphasis should be on respiratory and cardiovascular functioning and level of consciousness.

If the patient is comatose and can tolerate it, an endotracheal tube

should be passed. Cardiac status should be assessed, an intravenous catheter inserted, assisted respiration initiated if needed, and arterial blood
gasses monitored. Gastric lavage should be started and samples of gastric
contents, blood, and urine should be taken for toxicologic analysis.

As in the preceding circumstances, intensive care unit observation
should be maintained with respiratory and cardiovascular monitoring and
support. Conservative management with good nursing care gives the best
prognosis.

In all cases, once the crisis is past and the patient has become fully
conscious, he or she should be evaluated for appropriate medical detoxification or psychiatric aftercare.

Long-term Treatment

Because of the life-threatening nature of seizures connected with barbiturate withdrawal, it should be accomplished in an inpatient setting by
professionals who know what they are doing. All of the withdrawal syndromes related to barbiturates can be managed by detoxification with
phenobarbital, a long-acting barbiturate. In this program of treatment, 30
mg of phenobarbital is initially substituted for each hypnotic dose of the
individual's barbiturate of addiction. This phenobarbital stabilization period should continue for two days through peak liability, followed by
graded reduction of phenobarbital dosage over 7 to 20 days.

If the history of barbiturate abuse is variable or if the patient is using
multiple sedative-hypnotics, then a challenge of short-acting pentobarbital (100–200 mg) or of long-acting phenobarbital (100–200 mg) can be
used to test the individual's tolerance before starting the detoxification
schedule. A patient who does not have sedative-hypnotic tolerance will
respond to the challenge with signs of sedation, ataxia (inability to coor-
dinate voluntary body movements), and mild intoxication. One who has
developed tolerance will show minimal effect.

BENZODIAZEPINES

Chemical name: Chlordiazepoxide, clonazepam, clorazepate, diazepam, flurazepam, orazepam, oxazepam, prazepam, and triazolam

Category: Schedule IV

Product names: Ativan®, Centrax®, Librium®, Limbitrol®, Men-
rium®, Paxipam®, Serax®, Tranxene®, Valium®, Xanax®, etc.

Street names: Vitamin V and blues (both for Valium®)

Description: While the most familiar form of benzodiazepines is the small white (2 mg), yellow (5 mg), and blue (10 mg) Valium® tablet, these drugs come in a variety of tablet and capsule forms as well as injectable liquid form and in throwaway ampules.

Means of ingestion: Either swallowed in capsule or pill form or injected.

General Information

Benzodiazepines are currently the largest-selling drug group in the world. Their leading representative is Valium® (diazepam) the second most commonly prescribed single drug in the United States. Valium® is prescribed for the symptomatic relief of anxiety, insomnia, and muscle spasm. It is used in the treatment of convulsive disorders and alcohol dependency. The chemical structure, effects, and qualities of all benzodiazepines are similar, and these drugs, like barbiturates, can be discussed as a group.

Although there are risks involved in the medical use of benzodiazepines, they are safer than most other sedative-hypnotics, if managed correctly. They have a wide safety margin and less overdose potential than other drugs used for the same or similar purposes, such as the short-acting barbiturates.

Benzodiazepines are synthetic central nervous system depressants and sedative-hypnotics. They have similar qualities and effects to barbiturates and methaqualone and have a wide variety of therapeutic uses. They are a relatively new family of sedative-hypnotics that interact with specific benzodiazepine receptor sites in the brain. Among other effects, they produce anxiety relief without sedation at therapeutic doses. The first of these drugs, developed in the early 1960s, was chlordiazepoxide (Librium®). The next was diazepam (Valium®). Operating through receptor sites in the synaptic contact regions in the cerebral cortex, cerebellum, and hippocampus, these drugs work in part by relaxing the large skeletal muscles (Wesson & Smith, 1982).

In recent years, benzodiazepines — especially Valium® — have gained notoriety through media accounts of their effects both as a street drug and as prescribed medication. However, when prescribed and used judiciously, Valium® and the other benzodiazepines have an excellent therapeutic ratio with well-established therapeutic indications, relatively few side effects, and less overdose potential than most sedative-hypnotics.

Dangers

Benzodiazepines should not be taken if there is sensitivity to the other benzodiazepines or other sedative-hypnotics. They should not be taken by anyone with glaucoma, as they can increase interior eye pressure. They will cross the placental barrier and should not be used during pregnancy. They should *never* be used in conjunction with alcohol. Alcohol intensifies the toxic effects of benzodiazepines and greatly increases the possibility of dependence or of potentially fatal overdoses. There is also an additive effect with any other sedative-hypnotic.

Individuals with a personal or family history of alcoholism or drug addiction may have a predisposition to addiction and can develop dependence on benzodiazepines at therapeutic doses when taken daily for more than three months. Users taking more than therapeutic doses can develop dependency in a much shorter time. Individuals without a predisposition, however, can continue therapeutic dosages without developing dependence. Health professionals who prescribe benzodiazepines should learn how to diagnose potential dependence in a patient and how to recognize abuse (Smith, 1981).

We have recommended that physicians with patients on long-term benzodiazepine therapy give these patients periodic "holidays" from the drug at a graded reduction or zero dosage level for approximately seven days. This should be done approximately every 6 months, depending on patient needs. All benzodiazepines are cross-tolerant; that is, dependence on one automatically establishes dependence on all others. Consequently, switching a patient from one to another does nothing to solve dependency problems (Smith, 1979).

One thing a physician should definitely not do is to terminate benzodiazepine treatment abruptly. Abrupt withdrawal from these drugs, as from any sedative-hypnotic, can cause intense anxiety and agitation, withdrawal psychosis, and life-threatening seizures.

It should be noted that a rebound effect may accompany termination of benzodiazepine treatment — that is, the reemergence of symptoms that the drug was originally prescribed for, such as anxiety or agitation. The reemergence of these original symptoms can be mistaken for withdrawal symptoms.

Overdoses on benzodiazepines are less frequent than with other sedative-hypnotics, but they do occur. The symptoms are confusion, sleep or sleepiness, lack of response to pain, shallow breathing, lowered blood pressure, and coma.

Valium® has been used as a drug of deception. In several areas, counterfeit Quaaludes® or Mandrax® represented as having been smuggled in from Britain have proved to contain no methaqualone but instead high doses of Valium® (Renfroe, 1985). Habitual abusers of methaqualone say they can tell the difference in effect and do not like the counterfeits.

Emergency Treatment

A benzodiazepine overdose, especially if the drug has been taken in conjunction with alcohol or another sedative-hypnotic, is a life-threatening emergency. Treatment is the same as that for a barbiturate overdose and is covered extensively in the introductory section.

Long-term Treatment

The need for increasing amounts of benzodiazepines to achieve therapeutic effects is a sign of developing tolerance and dependence. If this or any subjective signs of habituation and dependence develop, detoxification from the drug should probably be undertaken. Under no circumstances should abrupt withdrawal after prolonged use, even at therapeutic doses, be attempted. Gradual reduction, or substitution and reduction of a slow-acting sedative-hypnotic such as phenobarbital, usually on an inpatient basis, is the safest way to detoxify. With diazepam (Valium®), the peak danger period for withdrawal seizure is 5 to 6 days into withdrawal.

Symptom reemergence should be managed by developing alternative symptom management programs that do not involve the taking of psychoactive substances.

METHAQUALONE

Chemical name: 2-methyl-3-(2-methylphenyl)-4 (3H)-quinazolinone

Category: Schedule II. No longer manufactured in United States.

Product names: Quaaludes®, Mandrax®, Melsedine®, Biphetamine-T® (in combination with amphetamine and dextroamphetamine), Mequin®, Parest®, Sopor®

Street names: Ludes, quackers, ducks, 714s, quas, quads, soapers, sopes

Description: Methaqualone occurs as a white, crystalline powder with a bitter taste. It is slightly soluble in water and freely soluble in alcohol. Its most common form in this country is in Quaalude®, which appears as flat white pills with LEMMON stamped in a semi-circle above the numbers 712 for the 150 mg size and 714 for the 300 mg size. Since production of Quaalude® ceased, most of these pills are counterfeit and contain drugs of deception.

Means of ingestion: Usually swallowed, but can be dissolved and injected or smoked in combination with marijuana. Abuse is often accompanied with ingestion of alcohol, with which it has a sedative-hypnotic additive effect.

General Information

Methaqualone is a quinazolinone, a nonbarbiturate sedative-hypnotic chemically similar to barbiturates and other sedative-hypnotics. Originally it was developed as an antimalaria drug. Its sedative-hypnotic qualities became apparent while it was being tested in India in the 1950s (Cohen, 1981). Although abuse of this drug had been reported in Japan and England, Quaalude® was approved for use in the United States in 1965 and placed on the federal Schedule V as a drug with minimum abuse potential. Quaalude® was then marketed by William H. Rorer, Inc. In the fall of 1978, production was taken over by the Lemmon Company.

Quaalude® was touted as a safe, effective, nonaddicting substitute for barbiturates. As such, it became America's sixth-best-selling sedative. It also did a brisk street business, because of its reputation as an aphrodisiac. This reputation was prompted by the disinhibiting effect methaqualone shares with all other sedative-hypnotics. There was no indication that it possessed any performance- or sensitivity-enhancing characteristics.

Fifteen years after it was first approved, methaqualone was moved from Schedule V to Schedule II. It had lost its status as a safe, nonaddicting sedative and become number three on the government's most abused drug list. In one year, methaqualone had been considered responsible for nearly 6000 emergency room visits and well over 100 overdose deaths in the United States alone.

The rise and fall of this drug has been more dramatic than most, but it has followed a pattern that is noticeable with opiates but most clear with sedative-hypnotics. With opiates, we saw the pattern in the development of heroin and may be seeing it in the evolution of methadone abuse. With sedative-hypnotics, time and again a new drug is discovered that counteracts tension and stress and produces euphoria, sedation and, a sense of well-being. Methaqualone, for example, was initially advertised as a "nonbarbiturate barbiturate," suggesting that it had all the advantages of the barbiturates but none of the disadvantages.

At first, the new drug is seen as an answer to the problems of tolerance, dependence, addiction, and adverse long-term side effects. In time, the bad news starts coming in, and yesterday's panacea becomes today's outlawed or controlled substance.

Perhaps any substance that produces these desired effects will prove in the long run to have a potential for overdose, dependence, addiction, and side effects. If that is the reality of the pharmacological situation, we may need to think more in terms of developing better control of the drugs we have rather than developing new ones that will merely perpetuate the cycle of tragedy we have already seen.

Recreational users of methaqualone describe the sensations it induces as "peaceful," "calm," "a rush," or like being drunk. They say that it produces a sense of well-being and sexual disinhibition.

Dangers

Use of methaqualone can cause headaches, hangovers, fatigue, dizziness, drowsiness, torpor, menstrual problems, loss of appetite, numbness, and pain in the extremities. Intoxication is similar to intoxication with any other sedative-hypnotic, including alcohol.

The overdose risk is high, especially when the drug is combined with alcohol. Overdose involves suppression of the cardiorespiratory systems and can be fatal.

Accidents can result from the impaired motor coordination of intoxication. One should never operate machinery or drive while high on methaqualone. Sexual performance, far from being enhanced, may be impaired by habitual high-dose use.

Methaqualone is especially dangerous when combined with alcohol in beverages or in over-the-counter medications, and it has a potentiating effect with any sedative-hypnotic. With frequent use, greater and greater quantities of the drug are needed to produce intoxication (tolerance develops). At the same time, the lethal dose remains relatively constant; thus, tolerance to methaqualone also increases the danger of a fatal overdose. Overdoses are marked by delirium, restlessness, hypertonia (excessive tension), muscle spasms, convulsions, coma, shock, respiratory arrest, and death.

There is a high risk of physical dependence, and withdrawal can be marked by insomnia, abdominal cramps, headache, anorexia, nightmares, delirium, and life-threatening convulsions and seizures (Smith et al., 1983).

Emergency Treatment

Overdose from methaqualone can be treated with immediate gastric lavage. It is a life-threatening situation and should be dealt with as an emergency. Spontaneous vomiting is common, and an airway needs to be maintained. General supportive measures should be undertaken. Extreme and prolonged convulsions may call for dialysis treatment.

Long-term Treatment

Withdrawal from methaqualone can be accomplished on an outpatient basis, but if 6 or more dosage units (pills) have been taken daily, the user should be hospitalized. As with other sedative-hypnotic dependencies, the usual treatment consists of substitution and step-down with a long-acting barbiturate and monitoring of vital signs to avoid life-threatening seizures.

Note: Counterfeit Methaqualone

In 1984 Lemmon, the sole United States manufacturer of Quaalude®, ceased production. Since that time, a high percentage of street Quaaludes®" are counterfeit and composed of drugs of deception.

Two major components in many of these pills are diazepam (Valium®) and phenobarbital, a long-acting barbiturate. Other ingredients have been the antihistamines pheniramine and doxylamine, the pain relievers aspirin and acetaminophen, and a "grab bag of miscellaneous additives including other barbiturates, arthritis medicines, O-toluidine (a toxic methaqualone precursor also used in manufacturing dyes) and epoxy glue" (Dye, 1983).

Obviously, these counterfeits pose a number of problems, not the least among them being the confusion caused in attempting to treat overdose and other adverse effects. Bogus ingredients can greatly affect the treatment of withdrawal symptoms. For example, with methaqualone withdrawal, the peak liability for seizures may be the second day. With high-dose diazepam, it occurs on the fifth to the seventh day, and if alcohol is involved, this peak can be delayed to the ninth or tenth day after abrupt cessation (Smith, 1984).

Interviews with the users of bogus methaqualone indicate that they do not get the same intense disinhibition/euphoria that they expect from methaqualone, and very often they complain of a prolonged drug effect like that of diazepam.

These look-alike methaqualones are appearing both in the form of Quaalude® Lemmon 714s and as British Mandrax®. With the latter, the pills are often represented as having been smuggled in from Europe or India. Mandrax®, as manufactured overseas, is a mixture of 250 mg of methaqualone and 25 mg of diphenhydramine hydrochloride, a potent antihistamine.

VOLATILE HYDROCARBONS

Category: Unscheduled commercial products

Product names: Toluene (plastic cement, airplane glue, lacquer thinner); xylene and acetone (fingernail-polish remover, model cement); gasoline; benzene (rubber cement, cleaning fluid, tube repair kits); naptha (lighter fluid); hexane (plastic cement); carbon tetrachloride (spot remover, dry cleaner); dichlorethylene and trichlorethylene (degreaser, dry cleaner, refrigerant, "liquid paper"); trichlormonofluoromethane and dichlordifluoromethane (aerosols and refrigerants)

Description: A variety of commercially available liquid solvents, gases and other volatile substances.

Means of ingestion: Sniffing (inhalation).

General Information

Inhalation of volatile substances to get high or to change consciousness goes back a long way. The classical Oracle at Delphi may have uttered her prophecies after inhaling gases that issued from the stones behind her throne (only the oracular priests could understand and interpret her incoherent comments). By the 19th century, such anesthetics as nitrous oxide and chloroform were sniffed recreationally, and ether-sniffing parties were common among students and physicians.

The current round of inhaling volatile substances began after World War II with airplane-glue sniffing. It expanded as American technology developed a wide range of hydrocarbon-based products, such as fast-drying glues and cements, paints, lacquers, varnishes, thinners, paint removers, and many aerosol-propelled products.

These substances are usually inhaled and are reported to give their users a feeling of well-being, reduced inhibitions, and mood elevation. In general, the effects are similar to those caused by alcohol and the other sedative-hypnotic drugs. At higher doses, users report effects similar to those found with nitrous oxide: laughing and giddiness, feelings of floating, dizziness, time and space distortion. Some of those substances are reported to produce hallucinations and psychedelic effects.

Most users of these substances are very young and have a low degree of drug sophistication. Usually they will sample whatever sniffable substance is in vogue at the time, but only once or twice, and then they will stop using it. Even chronic users usually "mature out of" the practice by their late teens.

Inhaling can be done either alone or in a group, although the deliriant nature of the high precludes much communication or interaction. The high usually lasts from 5 minutes to about an hour.

Dangers

Solvent sniffing can cause death by asphyxiation or suffocation, can impair judgment, and may produce irrational, reckless behavior. Abnormalities have occurred in liver and kidney functions. Bone marrow damage has occurred. Chromosome damage and blood abnormalities have been reported. Solvents have been cited as a cause of gastritis, hepatitis, jaundice, and peptic ulcers. Chronic users have developed slow-healing ulcers around the mouth and nose, loss of appetite, weight loss, and nutritional disorders. Irreversible brain damage has been reported.

The immediate negative effects are like those of being very drunk: Mental confusion, physical clumsiness, emotional confusion, and inability to think clearly are common. Outward early symptoms include dizziness, slurred speech, staggering, and drowsiness. Many of the injuries involved in the use of these substances result from reckless, irrational behavior and lack of good judgment. People intoxicated on inhalants are quite apt to have accidents and injure themselves or those around them. Driving or any use of machinery in this condition is very dangerous.

Many deaths attributed to solvent inhalants are caused by suffocation when users pass out with the plastic bags still glued to their noses and mouths. There is also a very real danger of death from acute solvent poisoning or aerosol inhalation. The mere provision of adequate ventilation and the avoidance of sticking one's head in a plastic bag are by no means sufficient safeguards against these dangers.

Brain, liver, kidney, and bone marrow damage in some users has been attributed to solvent sniffing, possibly because of hypersensitivity to these substances or chronic heavy exposure to them. At high doses, inhalants can cause rapid loss of control and loss of consciousness as well as potential overdose leading to irreversible damage to brain and body tissue or death from respiratory arrest (Wilford, 1981).

Other hazards include the possibility of freezing the larynx or other parts of the airway (particularly when refrigerants are inhaled) and potential spasms as these areas defrost. Blockage of the pulmonary membrane, through which oxygen is absorbed into the lungs, can occur. Death may also result from the ingestion of toxic ingredients along with the aerosol substance. The possibility is made more likely by the fact that commercial products not produced for human consumption are not required to list their ingredients on the label (Cohen, 1979).

Individual inhalants may have their own acute toxic reactions. These include gastric pain, headaches, drowsiness, irritability, nausea, mucous membrane irritation, confusion, tremors, nerve paralysis, optic nerve damage, vomiting, lead poisoning, anemia, and so on. The inhaling of aerosol fluorocarbons can cause "sudden-sniffing death" (SSD), wherein the heart is hypersensitized to the body hormone epinephrine, leading to a very erratic heartbeat, increased pulse rate, and cardiac arrest.

Tolerance and physical dependence have occurred among some chronic users. Withdrawal symptoms have included hallucinations, headaches, chills, delirium tremens, and stomach cramps. Alcohol and barbiturates may augment the adverse effects of high doses and of withdrawal (when alcohol or other drugs are used to mediate withdrawal).

Emergency Treatment

Acute reactions should be watched, and the sniffer should be prevented from self-harm. Bed rest and reassurance should be used rather than drugs or physical restraints. If the case is beyond that of mere acute intoxication, or if there is evidence of systemic poisoning, the sniffer should be taken to an emergency room or poison control center for long-term treatment.

Detoxification from chronic use should be monitored and withdrawal symptoms dealt with by a drug treatment program. The chronic user should be carefully informed of the dangers courted when one sniffs gases and inhalants.

MISCELLANEOUS SEDATIVE-HYPNOTICS

We have covered the most abused of the sedative-hypnotic type drugs individually and in depth. Here, we are reviewing several miscellaneous drugs in the general category in order to mention the specific aspects that may set them apart.

Chloral Hydrate (Cohidrate®, HS-Need®, Notec®, Orddrate®)

A Schedule IV sedative-hypnotic that predates the barbiturates, chloral hydrate was the Mickey Finn or "knockout drops" of old movies. It was used for such a purpose because a few drops, when mixed with alcohol, were very effective in causing sleep within an hour. As with any drug in this group, however, the additive combination was very dangerous. All the basic warnings and overdose/withdrawal treatment information general to sedative hypnotics applies. Chloral hydrate is most commonly prescribed as a daytime sedative or a sleeping medication and is sometimes used on an outpatient basis for the symptomatic treatment of opiate withdrawal (30 mg phenobarbital equals 250 mg chloral hydrate).

Ethchlorvynol (Placidyl®)

Ethchlorvynol is a Schedule IV sleeping medication. This drug is frequently used in suicide attempts and is not recommended for children under 15. Takes effect in 45 to 60 minutes and has a duration of 6 to 12 hours (30 mg phenobarbital equals 200 mg ethchlorvynol).

Glutethimide (Doriden®, Dormtabs®, Rolathimide®)

Glutethimide is a Schedule III sleeping medication. Is often mixed with codeine to produce a heroinlike high. In this form it is called "loads" or "setups." Glutethimide and codeine in this form have been responsible for several hundred overdose deaths in the United States since 1980. Glutethimide is also dangerous in its own right and is used in suicide attempts. All sedative-hypnotic precautions and treatments apply (30 mg phenobarbital equals 125 mg glutethimide).

Meprobamate (Arcoban®, Bamate®, Bamo 400®, Coprobate®, Equanil®, Evenol 400®, F.M. 400®, Kalmm®, Maso-Bamate®, Mepripam®, Meprocon®, Meprospan®, Meprotabs®, Meribam®, Miltown®, Neuramate®, Pax-400®, Protran®, Robam®, SK-Bamate®, Saronil®, Sedabamate®, Tranmep®)

Like **Tybamate** (Tybatran®), this drug is a carbamate. These drugs were the much publicized and often abused early "tranquilizers" of the post-World War II period. Miltown was often implicated in suicide attempts. Today, these drugs have largely been superseded medically by benzodiazepines.

These drugs are Schedule IV sedatives that are most frequently prescribed for anxiety and tension, often in combination with other substances. All precautions and warnings for benzodiazepines apply. Meprobamate is long-acting (30 mg phenobarbital equals 400 mg meprobamate).

Methyprylon (Noludarn®)

A Schedule III sleeping medication. All precautions regarding warnings and overdose/dependency treatment for sedative-hypnotics apply (30 mg phenobarbital equals 100 mg methyprylon).

General Anesthetics

Properly considered inhalants within the body of our inhalant subchapter, the general anesthetics deserve some mention of their own. As medical anesthetics, they occupy a unique place among inhalants. More than any other factor they may be responsible for the development of internal medicine as we know it, having facilitated our ability to perform complex surgical procedures without undue discomfort to the patient.

The three most common of these drugs are diethyl ether, chloroform and nitrous oxide. All three were abused recreationally before their medical facility was realized. Ether inhalation is still a periodic abuse pattern, but nitrous oxide is much more popular for recreational use.

Nitrous oxide is a sweet-smelling gas that is produced by heating ammonium nitrate. Medically it is used in dental procedures and other minor operations that require the patient to be conscious but temporarily sedated. Users have reported a variety of psychedelic experience with this gas, as well as loss of pain and feelings of exhilaration and euphoria. Onset is almost immediate, and these sensations end shortly after the supply is removed. In recreational use, balloons are often filled from tanks. Aerosol cans, in which a form of nitrous oxide is used as a propellant, may also be used. The drug itself is relatively safe if sufficient oxygen is taken with it. The greatest danger from its use is suffocation. Emergency treatment would include artificial respiration and cardiopulmonary resuscitation (CPR).

Central Nervous System Stimulants

HISTORICAL PERSPECTIVE

The spectre of massive stimulant abuse first struck the United States between 1968 and 1969. Amphetamine "epidemics" had earlier been reported in post-World War II Japan and in Sweden. In many ways, the abuse of amphetamines was a product of World War II, just as addiction to morphine followed America's Civil War. These stimulants were given liberally to pilots and combat troops, and after the war, production remained high.

Although high dose intravenous methamphetamine abuse decreased in the 1970s, medical indications for amphetamines and their production had both been significantly reduced by that time. Street use of oral amphetamines is still a major clinical concern, however.

In the late 1970s we encountered the recreational abuse of over-the-counter stimulants. These preparations are combinations of such legal ingredients as ephedrine, caffeine, and phenylpropanolamine. Sold as "pep pills" or "legal speed," these pills often resemble scheduled amphetamines and could be resold as the real thing.

Although cocaine has been around since the 19th century and was popularized by Sigmund Freud and by Arthur Conan Doyle's fictional detective Sherlock Holmes, its use remained esoteric until the 1970s. As late as 1979, many health professionals still considered cocaine a relatively benign drug. Since then, the picture has changed dramatically.

Most other medical stimulants are synthetic, but cocaine is a natural substance produced from leaves of the coca bush, growing in the uplands of South America. Used ceremonially by royalty and the priesthood in the pre-Columbian Inca civilization, coca leaves are still chewed for energy and as a dietary supplement. This use is indigenous to South American culture and is not considered abuse, but South American authorities are alarmed by the growing urban habit of smoking "pasta," a crude form of cocaine that produces effects similar to those of freebase smoking in the United States.

Cocaine hydrochloride, known on the street by such names as "coke," "blow," "snow," and "flake," usually appears as white crystalline flakes or powder that glitters. A recent development is "rocks," cocaine combined with a binding agent to form crystalline chunks measured to one-eighth to one-half gram in weight. The most common means of ingestion is insufflation (snorting) into the nasal membrane either from a small spoon or from a tube. These tubes can vary from rolled $100 bills to very fancy instruments. Cocaine is also dissolved in liquid and injected, smoked in unrefined forms such as "pasta," or further refined and smoked as "freebase."

Freebasing is an especially expensive and dangerous way of abusing cocaine. In this practice, the user further refines cocaine hydrochloride into a cocaine base with a low cooking point. The base is vaporized and the vapor inhaled. This vapor is then absorbed from the entire bronchial and lung surfaces, allowing great amounts of the drug to reach the brain very rapidly (Smith & Seymour, 1984).

Amphetamine in its pure form is a white crystalline material and is sold in this form as well as in tablet and capsule form. Amphetamine and amphetamine-like stimulants can be insufflated, imbibed in liquids, or swallowed in pills and capsules.

All chemical stimulants are related to epinephrine and norepinephrine. These are sympathomimetic amines (catecholamines) that occur naturally in the body. Stimulants are thought to work by either stimulating the production or inhibiting the re-uptake of these sympathomimetic amines in the central nervous system.

STIMULANT OVERDOSE AND ACUTE TOXICITY

The treatment of acute stimulant toxicity may vary according to the severity of symptoms, but it is basically the same. Toxic reactions are dose related and depend on a variety of factors including physical tolerance of the drug, psychological set, and sociocultural setting. These reactions can include psychological effects ranging from acute anxiety to full-blown stimulant psychosis with paranoia and auditory and visual hallucinations (Smith, 1984).

Acute toxicity symptoms tend to be similar no matter what stumulant may be involved: amphetamine, over-the-counter stimulants, or cocaine. We have recently encountered acute overdose toxicity with such psychedelic amphetamines as MDA or MDMA. The users present with anxiety, elevated pulse and heartbeat, and feelings of paranoia.

Deaths from Cocaine Toxicity

We have discovered in the treatment community that cocaine is a potent central nervous system stimulant, and like any psychoactive drug it has a pattern of use and abuse that is greatly influenced by sociocultural factors that include prevailing attitudes about the drug. Unfortunately, although we are recognizing the dangers of cocaine even with so-called recreational use, the public at large still considers it a relatively benign substance, and its use is currently widespread in the United States and spreading rapidly in other countries.

Recent statistics run counter to the belief that cocaine is a "safe" drug. The New York State Division of Substance Abuse Services reported in 1981 an increase in cocaine-related emergency-room deaths from 162 in the third quarter of 1978 to 518 in the third quarter of 1981. San Francisco reported a 300% increase in cocaine overdoses from 1980 to 1983, and similar reports have come in from across the United States.

In most of these fatal overdose cases, the cause of death has been cocaine-induced convulsions or cardiac arrythmias. While the majority of these deaths are a result of use by injection or freebase smoking, there has also been a substantial increase in deaths related to the insufflation or snorting of cocaine. Some deaths have resulted from "bodypacking." This is a means of smuggling wherein the courier swallows condoms filled with cocaine and carries these through customs in the stomach or intestinal tract. If one of these fragile containers bursts, the courier's body receives a massive overdose of cocaine.

Treatment of Acute Stimulant Toxicity

Acute stimulant toxicity can occur with any stimulant, including the two leading stimulants in our culture, caffeine and nicotine. However, most clinical cases involve amphetamines, amphetamine-like drugs, and cocaine.

Diagnosis of acute stimulant toxicity may be complicated by denial. Use of these drugs may be concealed by the client, in which case the cause of such abnormal behavior as acute agitation, anxiety, paranoia, or belligerent behavior may not be readily apparent.

Alternative diagnoses may include the following (Wesson & Smith, 1979):

- Paranoid schizophrenia
- Manic-depressive illness during the manic phase
- Psychoneuroses, especially anxiety neurosis and phobic states with panic
- Amphetamine-precipitated psychotic reaction
- Drug intoxication with psychedelics or phencylidine
- Hyperthyroid crises, including ingestion of thyroid preparation
- Pheochromocytoma

If the diagnosis is in doubt, history from friends or relatives can provide important clues. Urine testing may be inconclusive in that tests may show a false negative. This can be due to alkalinity, as urinary excretion is markedly reduced. Blood testing is the most helpful in confirming a diagnosis, but several days can elapse before results are available.

With stimulant overdoses, pupils are usually dilated, heart rate and blood pressure increased. Unfortunately, any psychological state that produces an epinephrine or norepinephrine response can also dilate pupils and increase heart rate and blood pressure.

If the client's behavior is not outside tolerable limits, and if blood pressure is not dangerously high, a period of observation is frequently helpful in establishing a correct diagnosis. Antipsychotic medication is effective in reducing agitated, hostile behavior but may further obscure the diagnosis, especially if toxicological analysis is not undertaken. For this reason, sedatives are initially preferred for behavioral control.

Time remains the most sure diagnostic proof. If the individual is suffering from amphetamine toxicity or cocaine toxicity, the abnormal behavior will subside in from 1 to 3 days as the level of stimulant in the blood falls. An individual who remains actively psychotic after this time and after urine stimulant levels are negative has a psychotic disorder instead of, or in addition to, an acute toxic stimulant reaction.

These latter cases may be stimulant-precipitated psychotic reactions. After a 24- to 48-hour observation and monitoring of blood levels, a diagnosis can usually be made. Clients suffering from a drug-precipitated psychotic reaction are usually hospitalized. Long-term maintenance with antipsychotic medication in conjunction with psychotherapy is the treatment of choice.

In many cases — including suicide attempts, accidental use by children, injection of unusually potent amphetamine or cocaine preparations, freebasing or bodypacking ruptures — massive overdoses may occur. In these instances, clients may be unconscious following seizures, hypertensive crises, or cerebrovascular accidents. In these cases, treatment strategies are usually determined on the basis of initial signs and symptoms. Strategies to reduce the amount of stimulant drug in the client's system include inducing emesis in conscious clients, gastric lavage with an acidic solution (ion trapping) in unconscious clients, and acidification of the urine with ascorbic acid or ammonium chloride to hasten excretion.

Hypertensive crises are treated with an alpha-adrenergic blocking agent such as phentolamine. The current antipsychotic drug of choice in treating stimulant toxicity is haloperidol.

Sufficiently large or prolonged doses of stimulants, including cocaine and methylphenidate (Ritalin), will induce a paranoid psychosis in anyone. However, unless the client suffers from schizophrenia, the psychotic reaction is dose dependent and will resolve as the stimulant is excreted from the body.

When stimulants are withdrawn from individuals who are dependent on them, a prolonged reaction takes place. These clients become depressed and anxious, and their sleep difficulties intensify. Clinical experience has demonstrated that these clients do not respond well to phenothiazine, lithium, or antidepressants and will often resume stimulant abuse (Seymour et al., 1982).

TREATMENT OF STIMULANT ADDICTION

The proliferation of what we can only call "cocaine addiction" in the last decade has changed the paradigm of addiction in the United States (Jellineck, 1960). Although a "disease concept" model was applied to alcohol in 1960, addiction to other drugs remained synonymous with physical dependence.

The paradigm of drug addiction led the general public, as well as many health professionals, to view cocaine as a relatively benign drug. Aside from producing episodic depression, anxiety, some sleep disorders, and a desire to return to use, stimulants were not thought of as producing a withdrawal symptomatology. Be that as it may, in the late 1970s and early 1980s, clinicians across the United States were inundated by cocaine users who found themselves incapable of getting off the drug. Curiously, many of these cocainists responded well to the twelve-step form of self-help and support treatment first developed for alcohol addicts by Alcoholics Anonymous.

As quantities of relatively potent cocaine at low prices have become available, the problem has intensified. Dealing with the problem has led to the following conclusions. Drug addiction is itself a pathological state characterized by compulsion, loss of control, and continued use despite adverse consequences. Physical dependence on a drug may contribute to addiction but is not synonymous with it. The causes of addiction are not yet fully known, but they appear to be a combination of genetic predisposition and sociocultural factors such as community attitudes and drug availability. Individuals who have parents or grandparents with drug or alcohol problems are much more at risk than those who do not. Although in some cases an underlying psychopathology may exist, in most cases addiction itself is a pathological state. In other words, there is no psychological profile of drug addicts—no character disorder that causes addiction.

Persons with the predisposition for addictive disease can go through life without ever knowing it, simply through abstention from psychoactive substances. Not all who use cocaine or other stimulants become addicted, but once addictive disease is in place, it is a pathological and deteriorating condition that will result in death if untreated.

Addiction is an incurable disease. There is, however, remission from this disease. Remission from active addiction is called "recovery" and depends on abstinence from all psychoactive substances.

Some individuals repeatedly become toxic with cocaine or other stimulants and demonstrate the inability to resist drug hunger. The greatest single reason why they relapse is the belief that they can return to controlled use of the cocaine. This ability is lost when the line into compulsive use is crossed.

A variety of treatment strategies have been implemented to facilitate the client's becoming drug free and entering into recovery. Withdrawal from stimulant dependence is characterized by depression, lethargy, and anxiety, which begin to resolve in about one week. Medication is rarely needed. Antidepressants should be employed only if an endogenous depression surfaces during the drug-free recovery period.

If the client has a secondary alcohol, sedative-hypnotic, or opiate dependence that poses a more serious withdrawal threat, specific detoxification medication in either the sedative-hypnotic or opiate drug group with gradual reduction is indicated.

Often, stimulant-dependent clients will be into an "upper/downer" abuse pattern, alternating their stimulant with an opiate or sedative-hypnotic. Amphetamine and cocaine abusers will mediate with barbiturates, alcohol, and heroin. Cocaine freebase smokers will often smoke high-potency Middle Eastern heroin to offset the "wired" effects of long-term stimulant abuse.

Once withdrawal is underway, recovery is best accomplished with a combination of individual and group therapy. A positive approach should be encouraged in contrast to "white-knuckle sobriety." This approach substantially requires educating the client on addictive disease in general and the principles of stimulant abuse specifically. Active allies including family are required, and the process is enhanced by family therapy. Long-term outpatient treatment should include a cocaine or amphetamine support group. Twelve-step programs such as Alcoholics Anonymous, Narcotics Anonymous, and Cocaine Anonymous have proved most helpful.

Exercise that produces cardiopulmonary stimulation in excess of 20 minutes at a time not only improves the client's physical state but actively reduces drug hunger as well.

The treatment process can be roughly divided into three phases: (1) establishing abstinence and sobriety, (2) developing a comfortable drug-free lifestyle, and (3) dealing with issues of arrested maturity and delayed withdrawal. Within a therapy group, one finds individuals in all stages. People whose recoveries are well established lend credibility to what is taught in the groups by showing their experience, while those in earlier stages help counteract the selective memory — i.e., euphoric recall of cocaine use—that often emerges after a period of abstinence (Ehrlich & McGeehan, 1985).

A subtle but powerfully evocative drug, cocaine is currently in the forefront as an addictive agent, although addiction to other stimulants can be a problem as well. Programs for treatment of cocaine dependence and addiction have appeared throughout the United States employing a variety of procedures. The treatment information we have shared in this article represents the most effective of these methods.

AMPHETAMINE

Category: Schedule II

Product names: Benzedrine®, Desoxyn®, Dexedrine®, Didrex®, Obetrol®, Eskatrol®, Biphetamine®, Amphaplex®, Delcobese®, Amphetamine sulfate®, Dexampex®, Ferndex®, Oxydess®, Robese®, Spancap®, Tidex®, Methampex®

Street names: Speed, uppers, pep pills, crank, bennies, dexies, meth, crystal, white crosses, black beauties, etc.

Description: In pure form, a white crystalline material. Sold as such as well as in tablets and capsules.

Means of ingestion: Amphetamine can be insufflated, imbibed in liquids, or injected. Most commonly, it is swallowed in pills or capsules.

General Information

Amphetamines are chemical stimulants that are related both chemically and pharmacologically to epinephrine and norepinephrine, sympathomimetic amines (catecholamines) that occur naturally in the body. They have been widely prescribed by physicians over the last 40 years for a variety of medical problems, including Parkinson's disease, depression, fatigue, sleep disorders, asthma, hyperactive behavior, and obesity (Smith & Seymour, 1980). Currently, they are approved medically only for the treatment of narcolepsy (attacks of deep sleep), hyperactivity in minimally brain-damaged children, and for short-term diet control in obesity. The ability of amphetamine to relieve sleepiness and fatigue and to increase short-term performance has led to extensive nonmedical use, particularly by people involved in activities that demand stamina and long periods of wakefulness: long-distance truck drivers, pilots, flight attendants, and entertainers. In wartime, amphetamines have been supplied in quantity to pilots and combat troops. They have also been commonly used by students cramming for exams, and by athletes to enhance their performance.

These drugs have also been heavily abused for their rush and their euphoric effect at high injected dosages. Japan, Sweden, and the United States have all experienced epidemics of high-dose intravenous methamphetamine abuse (Smith & Wesson, 1973).

The pharmacological effects of amphetamines include cardiovascular stimulation, central nervous system stimulation, increased body temperature, and appetite suppression. These physical symptoms are often accompanied by a feeling of well-being. High-dose intravenous use produces a euphoria that comes on with a rush highly prized by users. The euphoria produced by these drugs is caused by their stimulation of mood-elevating chemicals in the brain such as epinephrine and norepinephrine (Seymour et al., 1982). Amphetamines may also give their users a sense of false courage by inhibiting MAO (monoamine oxidase), the overproduction of which is known to produce neurotic fears.

In the United States, the high-dose intravenous methamphetamine epidemic peaked in 1969. Its decline has been attributed to realistic drug education in the street and the obviously dire physical effects of long-term high-dose abuse. The abuse of amphetamines in oral dosages continued to be widespread on into the 1970s. In that decade, however, the manufacturers, in cooperation with the Drug Enforcement Administration and the Federal Food and Drug Administration took measures to decrease diversion for nonmedical use. These measures included a drastic reduction in the amount of amphetamine produced in this country. At the same time, medical uses of these drugs were limited to the indications listed above. Any other medical use must be considered experimental. Most amphetamine preparations were also made Schedule II controlled substances at that time, requiring triplicate prescriptions and enforcement surveillance. As a consequence of these actions, there is now very little "real" amphetamine on the street. Over 90% of street amphetamines are actually look-alike pills that use such legal stimulants as caffeine, ephedrine, and phenylpropanolamine to produce something vaguely resembling an amphetamine effect.

Dangers

Prolonged high-dose use of amphetamines, particularly if accompanied by sleep deprivation, will produce an amphetamine psychosis that resembles paranoid schizophrenia — the user becomes very frightened and out of touch with reality. Prolonged use can also contribute to malnutrition and a weakening of the immune system. Injection of amphetamine also exposes the user to needle diseases such as hepatitis and endocarditis. Injection can also expose the user to acquired immune deficiency disease (AIDS).

Amphetamines elevate blood pressure and can cause a variety of medical crises including heart attacks and strokes. Diet preparations that contain both amphetamines and thyroid extracts should be avoided since, when combined, they elevate blood pressure to dangerous levels. Even at low doses, the effect of amphetamine on the user's body temperature can provoke heat stroke in hot weather if the user engages in physical exertion.

Individuals can "overamp." An overamped person is conscious but unable to move or speak. The condition is also characterized by rapid pulse, elevated temperature, increased blood pressure, and breathing distress.

Sexually, orgasm and ejaculation may be delayed at high doses, or sexual interest may disappear completely (Cohen, 1981).

Withdrawal from amphetamine dependence is not characterized by seizures but can produce severe depression.

Emergency Treatment

A massive stimulant overdose constitutes a medical emergency and requires immediate professional attention. Seizures and cardiac arrhythmias may call for medication. Anxiety reactions can be managed by reassurance and, occasionally, sedative-hypnotic medication.

Victims of massive overdose may be unconscious following seizures and may have hypertensive crises or even cerebrovascular accidents. Treatment strategies are largely determined by the initial signs and symptoms. Strategies to reduce the amount of amphetamine in the system include inducing emesis in conscious victims, gastric lavage with an acidic solution (ion trapping) in unconscious individuals, and acidification of the urine with ascorbic acid or ammonium chloride to enhance excretion. Hypertensive crises are treated with an alpha-adrenergic blocking agent such as phentolamine. The current drug of choice in treating amphetamine toxicity is haloperidol.

Long-term Treatment

Stimulant psychoses usually begin to fade once the drug has metabolized. When amphetamines are withdrawn, these clients become depressed and anxious. Their sleep difficulties intensify. It is important to distinguish carefully between acute toxic reactions that are dose related and drug-precipitated psychotic reactions that continue after blood and urine tests are negative for amphetamines. Usually a period of observation of 1 or 2 days may be necessary to distinguish between the two conditions. In the latter cases, psychiatric hospitalization and antipsychotic medication may be required.

Long-term treatment for recovery from amphetamine addiction usually involves drug counseling on an outpatient basis with an emphasis on abstinence. In cases where drug hunger is too strong to combat on an outpatient basis, longer-term modified medical model aftercare centers may be considered (Smith et al., 1978; Smith et al., 1979).

CAFFEINE

Category: Ingredient in many legal substances and over-the-counter drugs

Product names: Coffee, tea, guarana, maté, cola, chocolate, cocoa, etc.

Street names: Many, occurring in virtually all cultures. The names for coffee alone are legion.

Description: Caffeine is rarely seen in its pure, chemical form. As an ingredient in over-the-counter preparations, it appears in a variety of pills and capsules. It has also gained some notoriety in look-alikes and drugs of deception in which it is mixed with such substances as phenylpropanolamine and ephedrine in pills, capsules, and powders designed to resemble cocaine or scheduled stimulants.

Most commonly, caffeine is the intrinsic psychoactive ingredient in a variety of stimulant drinks and foods. These are usually bitter and are mixed with sugar or other sweetening agents to make them potable.

Means of ingestion: Products containing caffeine may be insufflated as a powder, swallowed as pills or capsules, sipped as beverages, or eaten.

General Information

Caffeine is one of the xanthines, a group of effective and potent stimulants. All caffeine-based preparations, with the possible exception of chocolate, are used primarily for their stimulant qualities. Little is known about coffee pharmacology.

Caffeine was first isolated from coffee in 1821. Coffee, however, seems stronger in psychoactive properties than caffeine alone would provide (Weil & Rosen, 1983). Coffee originated in Ethiopia, where the crushed beans were molded into a ball with fat to provide a day's ration for nomads in need of quick energy. Coffee use then spread to Arabia, where it was used in religious ceremonies (Farb & Armelagos, 1980). Many cultures use other caffeine-active stimulants. England and the Far East use tea, which has a caffeine potency comparable to coffee's but not as much stimulant effect. Brazilians use guarana, their national drink made from the seeds of a jungle tree. Argentina has maté. East Africans chew kola nuts – and nearly everyone drinks Coca-Cola or its analogues. Then there is chocolate . . .

Dependence on coffee is very common in Western society. It is so thoroughly approved as a stimulant that most people who use it regularly are surprised to learn that it is indeed a drug.

Coffee is usually prepared by grinding or crushing the toasted beans and leaching the caffeine and flavor elements from them with hot water or steam. The result is a bitter brown liquid that may have milk added to precipitate some of the acids and sugar added to sweeten the taste and provide an additive stimulant effect.

Coffee is nearly ubiquitous in our culture. Many people drink it after or during every meal. Businesses have regular "coffee breaks." It is used as a social lubricant, especially when alcohol is inappropriate. In Europe, many people while away their time, either alone or in groups, sipping coffee in cafes – which are named for the beverage.

American coffee, except for the brew served at truck stops and in New Orleans, has traditionally been weak and insipid. In recent years, stronger strains such as "dark French roast" and such preparations as espresso, cafe Greque, and Turkish coffee have appeared here. In parts of Florida, businessmen are reportedly gulping espresso-type "Cuban" coffee by the mugful.

Dangers

Caffeine is addictive. Excessive coffee drinking is characterized by all three addiction indicators: compulsion, loss of control, and continued use despite adverse consequences. There is even evidence of a physical withdrawal syndrome (Goldstein et al., 1965). Excess caffeine intake can exacerbate recovery from drugs and alcohol by increasing anxiety, depression, and insomnia. High doses of caffeine, the equivalent of 8 to 12 cups of coffee, can produce anxiety, nervousness, irritability, tremulousness, muscle twitchings, insomnia, sensory disturbances, hyperventilation, rapid heart beat, irregular heart beat, flushing, increased urination and genitourinary inflammation, and gastrointestinal disturbances. Recent studies indicate that in people afflicted with addictive disease or high sensitivity to stress and anxiety, these symptoms occur at levels equivalent to 1 or 2 cups of coffee a day (Whitfield, ms).

There has been some concern about the possible involvement of caffeine in reproductive abnormalities. Both animal and human studies indicate that women should avoid heavy caffeine use during pregnancy. These studies have shown that use of caffeine in amounts equivalent to eight or more cups of coffee a day is related to an increased incidence of spontaneous abortions and stillbirths, breech deliveries, and cyanosis at birth. If the usual safety precautions respecting drugs were adopted with respect to caffeine, bags of coffee would be required to bear a label warning pregnant women to consume no more than a small fraction of a cup each day (Addiction Research Foundation, 1981).

Millions of people in the United States are mildly addicted to coffee. This condition is usually ignored or overlooked until one tries to stop. Withdrawal symptoms can appear after stopping as little as a two-cup-a-day habit. Symptoms can include lethargy, irritability, disorientation, working difficulty, constipation, and a general to intense headache. These symptoms decrease rapidly and are usually gone within three days. It should be noted that all preparations containing caffeine have an additive effect—while reducing coffee intake, some people continue to ingest large quantities of soft drinks; tea; chocolate; and caffeine-based cold, allergy, or weight-reduction pills.

Emergency Treatment

Treatment often takes the form of reassurance that the overdose symptoms are not a heart attack or some other life-threatening event. The victim should rest if possible and let the symptoms pass. Sedative hypnotics should not be used to counteract the symptoms of a caffeine overdose. By the same token, coffee and other caffeine preparations should not be used to counter the effects of alcohol. All this does is produce a most undesirable presence, the wide-awake drunk.

Long-term Treatment

Anyone who suffers from caffeine overdoses may need to quit. Also, many general physical complaints are possibly the result of too much caffeine. The drug is so ubiquitous that complete avoidance of it is all but impossible. It is possible, though, to check overall caffeine intake, including pills and soft drinks, and to try for a lower overall consumption level. A major step in this direction involves coffee intake. Fortunately, with the increasing awareness in our culture of the adverse effects of caffeine, better-tasting preparations of decaffeinated coffee and tea are becoming available as alternatives. Recovering addicts should moderate or stop their caffeine intake. Fortunately, the dependence on coffee often ends with the three-day withdrawal.

CHOCOLATE

Chemical name: Theobroma cocao (food of the Gods)

Category: Not scheduled. Readily available over the counter.

Product names: Cocoa, hot chocolate, chocolate chips, kisses, syrup, a variety of bars usually with a trade name, pudding and pie.

Street names: Candy, pogy bait, brown speed, etc.

Description: Comes in liquid or solid form ranging in color from a creamy white to a dark brown. Powdered form usually cocoa colored but may range to dark brown in some cases.

Means of ingestion: Powdered form is usually mixed with liquid, often either water or milk, and sipped either hot or cold. Liquid syrup may be poured over ice cream or mixed into ice cream soda drinks and eaten. As a solid, it may be formed into bars of solid chocolate, used to coat various candy fillings in bars or bon-bons (bonbon means good twice over), mixed with nuts and other ingredients to make fudge, baked into cookies or coated with a hard sugar protective layer in small lozenges that "melt in your mouth, not in your hand." Melted chocolate may be used to coat nuts, fresh strawberries, and other fruit, and to ice cakes. In Europe a spreadable form, usually mixed with ground chestnuts, is spread on bread. In most cases chocolate is eaten or drunk. We know of no instances where chocolate has been either insufflated or injected.

General Information

Chocolate is made from the seeds of the cacao tree, a wide-branching evergreen that grows near the Equator. Although the tree originated in Mexico and Central America, it is now grown in Africa and parts of Asia as well. The seeds, which appear in large pods directly from the tree's trunk and branches, are called cacao beans. These beans have a high fat content which is known as cacao butter. Sometimes this butter is used as a confection called "white chocolate" or as an ingredient in suntan lotion. Most often, however, it is mixed with chocolate as a binding agent.

When the beans are defatted and ground into a powder, the result is cocoa. In the United States, this powder is mixed with hot milk and sugar. This hot cocoa is a mild stimulant wherein the additive effect of the stimulant sugar is probably mediated to some degree by the sedative L-tryptophan in the hot milk. The resulting beverage is considered "safe for children." In that it resembles creamed coffee, it can be given to children as an alternative to coffee. Adults sometimes mix cocoa and coffee for an even greater stimulant effect for themselves although this practice is not widespread.

This drug was used ceremonially and as a stimulant in pre-Columbian Mexico, where it was prepared for the rulers and priests in an elaborate ritual. Mexican hot chocolate remains quite distinctive. It has a higher cocoa-butter content than others and is mixed with flavorings such as cinnamon and ground almonds and packed into wheel-shaped bricks. These bricks are broken into clay pots of hot milk and the mixture is whipped until frothy with decorated wooden paddles spun between the palms. On market days, the sun rises to charcoal fires with frothing chocolate being spun over them.

In the Basque north-coastal states of Spain, a chocolate is brewed that is as strong and dark and thick as chocolate syrup. In cafes along the esplanade in San Sebastian, this concoction is sipped very hot because the viscosity drops as it cools to a consistency similar to chocolate mousse. The stimulant potency of this drink is startling.

Eating chocolate is made by adding cocoa butter back into the ground and roasted beans. A lot of ingenuity goes into this process, creating many distinctive kinds of chocolate with a great range of quality rivaling that of fine wines. The competition is great.

The psychoactive ingredient in chocolate is caffeine, one of the xanthines, a group of effective and potent stimulants that also inhabit tea and coffee.

Chocolate is usually considered a food rather than a drug. Although its stimulant qualities do contribute much of its appeal, it is probably the only stimulant that can cause weight gain rather than weight loss. Aside from its caffeine content, little is known about chocolate pharmacology. Some recent studies have linked enzymes that appear in the metabolization of chocolate with those reported to be present in persons in love. This contention is sure to give rise to much future speculation in the field.

Dangers

Caffeine is addictive, and chocolate has as much of an addiction potential as coffee or any other caffeine preparation. People who regularly consume chocolate or go on chocolate-eating binges may not realize that they are involved with a drug, but their consumption usually follows the same sort of pattern as with coffee, tea, and cola drinks.

Some people have or develop allergies to chocolate which produce a wide variety of physical symptoms. The most common of these are dermatological or digestive. Overdoses are very rare, but they do occur. Symptoms can include anxiety, nervousness, tremulousness, muscle twitching, insomnia, sensory disturbances, hyperventilation or rapid heavy breathing, rapid heartbeat, irregular heartbeat, flushing, increased urination, and gastrointestinal disturbances.

Many general physical complaints can result from too much caffeine. Coffee, tea, diet pills, cola drinks, and cold medications all contain this drug, and the effects are additive. People are rarely aware of how much caffeine they may be ingesting on a regular basis.

Emergency Treatment

Chocolate overdose can be treated symptomatically and as any mild stimulant overdose. In that a small bar of chocolate contains about 20 mg of caffeine or about a fifth of the amount in a cup of coffee, the need for emergency treatment seems highly unlikely.

Long-term Treatment

Symptoms of withdrawal from caffeine do occur and may include some lethargy, irritability, disorientation, working difficulty, and headaches. With chocolate these symptoms should be minor. If they do occur, they decrease rapidly and are usually gone within a few days.

Someone who is consuming too many caffeine-containing products should try alternatives. Decaffeinated coffees and teas are available in increasing variety and quality. There are noncaffeinated soft drinks, and chocolate substitutes such as carob that do not contain caffeine.

COCAINE HYDROCHLORIDE

Chemical name: 2-beta-carbomethoxy-3-beta-benoxytropane

Category: Schedule II

Product names: Cocaine Hydrochloride Topical Solution®

Street names: Coke, snow, lady, blow, gold dust, Bernice, she, damablanca, flake, pasta, freebase, rock, etc.

Description: Cocaine usually appears as white crystalline flakes or powder that glitters. Two recent developments are "rock," cocaine combined with a binding agent to form crystalline chunks usually one-eighth to one-half gram in weight, and "crack," an illicit street-sale form of cocaine freebase made with baking soda.

Means of ingestion: The most common means of ingestion is insufflation or snorting up into the nasal mucosa. Classically this is done with a rolled-up, new hundred-dollar bill, but a variety of instruments may be used ranging from the pocket clip of a ballpoint pen cap to highly ornate tiny spoons made of precious substances. The cocaine may be scooped from a container with these spoons or chopped (powdered with the edge of a razor or knife blade) and spread into lines on a smooth surface, often a mirror or polished stone.

The drug may also be dissolved in liquid and injected, smoked in an unrefined form as "pasta," or further refined and smoked as "freebase."

General Information

Cocaine is an alkaloid refined from the leaves of *Erythroxylum coca* and several other species of coca shrubs that grow in the highlands of Peru, Bolivia, and Colombia as well as in the Amazon Basin. Indians in these regions have chewed coca leaves since pre-Columbian times, when they were reserved for Inca royalty. For hundreds of years, however, they have been used to facilitate work performance and as a dietary supplement in the harsh South American uplands.

In making cocaine hydrochloride, the coca leaves are placed in gasoline drums and saturated with kerosene. They are mashed, and the macerated leaves are then subjected to sulfuric acid to release the cocaine "pasta." This paste is the raw material that by itself can be — and is — smoked in South American urban centers. This pasta is further refined through solvent extraction into the cocaine hydrochloride that is shipped to the United States. Because its bulk is the same or a little less than cocaine hydrochloride, the drug is increasingly being shipped in pasta form and refined here in the States.

In 1860, Albert Niemann of Göttingen, Germany, first isolated cocaine from the leaf and noted its numbing effect on the tongue (Gay, 1981). For the rest of the century a number of famous physicians, including Sigmund Freud, experimented with cocaine. Its use in "tonics" and patent medicine was widespread. Coca-Cola, which was first sold as a tonic, still uses coca leaves — with the cocaine removed — for flavoring. By 1899, cocaine abuse was being recognized and publicly acknowledged. A political note entered when cocaine prohibitionists launched a campaign of fear of "cocaine-crazed black dope fiends" to gain their ends. In 1914, cocaine was included as a narcotic in the Harrison Act, and its recreational use went underground.

The effects of cocaine include localized numbing of the nose, gums, and throat, and feelings of euphoria and calm alertness, along with an overblown sense of one's physical and mental abilities. A potent central nervous system stimulant, cocaine affects the neurotransmitters norepinephrine and dopamine. As a result, heart rate increases; pupils dilate;

blood sugar rises; blood vessels constrict, increasing the flow to the brain and muscles; sphincters tighten; digestion slows; and body temperature rises.

At low doses, cocaine enhances sexual desire and tactile awareness. At high doses and over time, however, it impairs sexual performance. It is often used in combination with other drugs such as alcohol or other sedative-hypnotics or with heroin in an upper/downer cycle of abuse. Injected with heroin the mixture is called a "speedball" and can have highly deleterious effects.

Medical use of cocaine is currently limited to topical anesthesia and, in a modified Brompton's solution (containing methadone, cocaine, and alcohol), for treatment of pain in terminal cancer patients. Its use has been suggested for the treatment and diagnosis of certain mental disorders (Smith & Wesson, 1978; Grinspoon & Bakalar, 1976).

Dangers

Until fairly recently, cocaine was considered a relatively benign drug. Because of its vasoconstrictive (blood-vessel constricting) effect on the nasal capillaries, insufflation was considered to be self-limiting at a "safe" level. Cocaine travels through these capillaries to the heart, through the lungs, back to the heart, and then to the brain and other organs. Its lack of a physical withdrawal symptomatology as compared with alcohol, other sedative-hypnotics, and opiates such as heroin was cited as indicating that cocaine was not an addictive drug. Further, many of its users were the young go-getters of our society who saw the drug as an aid in both their business and social life. The continuation of the myth is perhaps one of cocaine's greatest dangers in that it promotes denial of the drug's disabling and addictive character and keeps people who truly need treatment from seeking it.

Because cocaine does constrict the blood vessels of the nasal mucosa, prolonged use can cause irritation and eventually necrosis (tissue death). This effect has been disproportionately stressed in street mythology, however, and perforated septums are rare. More common is chronic redness and rhinitis (runny nose).

Although they are more common from the injection or smoking of cocaine, fatal overdoses from insufflation are on the increase as well. The mechanism of death in most of these overdose reactions is either cocaine-induced convulsions or toxic heart reactions brought on by depression of the medullary centers (Smith, 1983).

Rupture of containers for smuggling of cocaine in the gastrointestinal system has also resulted in death from massive overdose.

Means of ingestion: The freebase is heated in a retort, foil, or other container and the vapor is inhaled as the freebase vaporizes.

General Information

Cocaine freebase is the alkaloidal base of cocaine hydrochloride, which in turn is a refined extract of the coca plant leaves. Coca has been cultivated since ancient times in the uplands of South America, where the leaves are chewed for their mild stimulant and euphoric effects. Coca should not be confused with cacao, the Central American bush from which cocoa and chocolate are produced. Both do have stimulant qualities.

The primary method of cocaine use in the United States has been through nasal insufflation, i.e., snorting. Absorption through the nasal mucosa is limited, however. Not only is the nasal surface small, but the vasoconstrictive property of cocaine shrinks the capillaries that carry the cocaine into the system. For these reasons, cocaine use has been commonly viewed as relatively benign. With the dramatic increase we have seen in cocaine addiction in recent years and the increase in cocaine-related medical emergencies, the view that cocaine is relatively free of serious health consequences or dependence liability looks more like a case of professional and public wishful thinking.

In recent years, the smoking of cocaine freebase has become increasingly popular even though it is very, very expensive. Freebase kits used for the home conversion of the hydrochloride are readily available.

The idea of smoking coca products is not new. F. R. Jeri of Peru visited the Haight-Ashbury Free Medical Clinic in 1977 and reported that the smoking of cocaine paste was the greatest drug problem in his country. Urban Peruvians smoke coca paste (pasta) — a crude extract of coca leaves containing coca sulfate, ergonine, other coca alkaloids, benzoic acid, and kerosene residue — in tobacco or marijuana cigarettes (Jeri et al., 1978). The discovery that a small number of cocaine abusers were freebasing came as a result of this disclosure. In fact, freebase may have been discovered in the United States as a result of a misunderstanding of what was being practiced in Peru. Drug chemists misinterpreted the word "pasta" or "basa" to mean "base" or alkaline refined for a nonacetic cocaine formation that could be smoked.

Smoking of cocaine hydrochloride is occasionally reported in the United States, but in this form cocaine's melting point is 197°C and most of it is burned without effect. Conversely, freebase melts at 98°C and vaporizes easily.

Because the freebase is absorbed directly into the lungs, much higher dosages are possible than with insufflation and they are much more rapidly effective than with injection. Users describe numbing of the mouth and throat and an intense euphoric "rush." The euphoria is quickly followed by irritability. During this phase, users feel compelled to "do more freebase" (Wesson, 1979).

Dangers

In addiction-prone individuals, snorting cocaine can become compulsive, with loss of control and continued use despite obvious adverse consequences. The probability of cocaine dependence is increased with freebasing while the cost factor is multiplied. Illicit cocaine hydrochloride is expensive as is. When this street drug is further refined to make freebase, the cost can become astronomical. Fortunes have been spent on this practice.

Owing to cocaine's local anesthetic properties on the bronchial mucosa, irritation is not noticed during use. Post-use bronchial irritation may last several days. Bronchitis can be severe, with chronic users coughing up blood and black-streaked sputum for weeks following sustained use. Unlike snorting, in which the constriction of blood vessels in the nose decreases absorption with continuing use, freebasing utilizes the bronchial mucosa, which remains a large, efficient absorption surface. This greatly increases the risk of cocaine overdose.

With the massive dosages made possible by freebase smoking, drug-induced psychosis and various physical complications can occur. Users have become physically emaciated and psychologically devastated by high-dose, daily use.

Both ethyl ether and petroleum ether, which are used in the refining of freebase, are extremely flammable. Individuals have been severely burned while preparing freebase with these substances.

Finally, some cocaine users employ sedatives, including alcohol or opiates, simultaneously or sequentially with freebasing to combat the "over-amped" feeling produced by the cocaine. This practice may cause secondary drug dependence of the opiate or alcohol type.

Emergency Treatment

Overdoses on cocaine freebase can range from anxiety to seizure. With over-amp anxiety reaction, all that is necessary is reassurance and sedative hypnotic medication such as diazepam (Valium®) if indicated. Medical life support measures and intravenous diazepam are necessary for lifethreatening, cocaine-induced seizures. The cocaine-induced psychosis that occurs after a long run of freebasing usually requires hospitalization and antipsychotic medication such as haloperidol.

Long-term Treatment

Although cocaine does not have a recognized physical withdrawal syndrome, cocaine addicts do fit within the behavioral symptomatology of addictive disease – i.e., compulsion, loss of control, and continued use despite adverse consequences. Hunger for the drug runs high both during and after detoxification, and cocaine addicts often need inpatient treatment to keep them from finding and using more of the drug.

Freebasers and cocaine addicts in general respond well to such self-help treatment modalities as Alcoholics Anonymous and peer support groups. Abstinence and recovery are the key. Cocaine treatment programs with a recovery theme are becoming widespread but an AA chapter that will accept cocaine users is also effective.

TOBACCO

Category: Some states have age restrictions on retail purchase of tobacco.

Product names: Generally classified as cigarettes, cigars, pipe tobacco, snuff, chewing tobacco, and roll-your-own. Each of these have a number of competitive brand names.

Street names: Sot weed, coffin nails, butts, squares, smokes, fags, stogies, cancer sticks, chawbaccy, cheroots, etc.

Description: Tobacco is commercially produced as a large leaf, usually tan to dark brown in color. This is usually cut into thin strips, shredded, or flaked for consumption. *Cigarettes* are usually cylinders of shredded tobacco wrapped in a single tube of thin, chemically treated white paper. Some brands have filters on one end that are composed of cellulose, charcoal, cotton filaments, or some other porous but absorbent substance. The purpose of these filters is to trap some of the less desirable tars and other carcinogens that are found in tobacco smoke.

Cigars are usually composed of a more coarsely cut, more potent tobacco and are wrapped in tobacco leaf rather than paper. They range in size from slightly larger than king-size cigarettes to nearly a foot in length and an inch or so in diameter.

Pipe tobacco is also rough cut and usually aromatic.

Snuff is either flaked or powdered and usually comes in small tins.

Chewing tobacco is dark and somewhat oily in appearance, made up of larger leaf pieces and compressed into small cakes. In appearance they look somewhat like miniature marijuana "kilo bricks."

Roll-your-own usually comes in small pouches or larger round tins and is sold along with packs of cigarette papers.

Means of ingestion: Cigarettes and cigars are placed with one end in the mouth and the other end is lighted. The user draws the smoke through the length by puffing in. The smoke of cigarettes is usually inhaled, while that of cigars is not.

Pipe tobacco is artfully packed into a variety of pipes. These instruments usually have a bowl for the tobacco that is connected to a hollow stem that the smoker grips in the mouth and puffs through. The pipe bowls may be made from a variety of materials including clay, cancerous growth from trees (burls), and dried corncobs. When tobacco first became popular in Europe after the "discovery" of America, innkeepers kept clay pipes with very long stems for their guests. As a hygienic measure, each smoker snapped a small piece from the end of the pipestem before using it. As with cigars, the smoke of pipes is rarely inhaled directly into the smoker's lungs. This privilege is reserved for others in the same room.

A pinch of snuff is usually placed between gum and lip, and its pychoactive ingredients are leached into the system through the mucosa. Tobacco chewers bite off a wad from their cake and chew it. As these forms of unsmoked tobacco irritate the salivary glands, users of snuff and chewing tobacco tend to spit or expectorate a lot.

General Information

Tobacco was used ceremonially in pre-Columbian America for over 2000 years. Its use was carried to Europe by early explorers. In fact, Sir Walter Raleigh may have sent the first boatload of tobacco across the Atlantic. Tobacco's active ingredient, nicotine, acts by stimulating and blocking certain receptor sites, chemical receptors in some arteries, and thermal and pain receptors in the skin and tongue. It also increases electrical activity in parts of the brain.

Use of this highly controversial drug was denounced by both church and state. It was forbidden in 17th century England, and at times, conviction for selling it carried a death penalty.

Nicotine is absorbed through the entire respiratory tract, the oral and nasal mucosa, the gastrointestinal tract, and even the skin. Up to 90% of inhaled nicotine is absorbed by the lungs. Nicotine is a highly toxic poison and has been used as an insecticide.

Like PCP (phencyclidine), tobacco can act as both a stimulant and a depressant. It can increase respiration, heart rate, and blood pressure while decreasing appetite. Tobacco intoxication is characterized by euphoria, lightheadedness, giddyness, dizziness, elevated heartbeat and respiration, and a tingling sensation in the extremities. However, this intoxication is usually only noticed in beginning tobacco users. Both tolerance and dependence develop rapidly, and the "high" gets lost in the shuffle. Chronic users usually stabilize their intake at some point in their addiction into something that resembles a maintenance dosage.

Because nicotine is a vasoconstrictor, cigarettes have sometimes been used to reduce bleeding of battlefield wounds.

Dangers

It has been said that tobacco in the form of machine-made cigarettes is the most addictive substance on earth. Nearly everyone who starts smoking becomes addicted. Withdrawal symptoms include nervousness, restlessness, sleep disturbance, sweating, reduced heart rate and blood pressure, inability to concentrate, compulsive eating, headaches, and severe irritability. The nicotine craving, or drug hunger, may continue for life.

Overdoses usually occur before tolerance sets in and are not considered serious. Symptoms include dizziness, nausea, and difficulty in breathing. This syndrome should not be confused with acute nicotine poisoning in which concentrations of nicotine have been absorbed. Nicotine poisoning is usually the result of accidental ingestion or absorption of nicotine-based insecticides, suicide attempts, or certain misguided and highly dangerous folk medicine "cures." Acute nicotine poisoning is serious and should be dealt with on an emergency basis (Manguerra & Freeman, 1982-83).

Most of the adverse effects of tobacco result from long-term, chronic use. These include heart disease, obstructive pulmonary and bronchial disease, cancer, noncancerous mouth disease, gum and jawbone deterioration, gastrointestinal disease, anorexia and eating disorders, and allergic reactions. Recent studies indicate that use of smokeless tobacco — i.e., snuff and chewing tobacco — can be just as dangerous as smoking and a cause of mouth and throat lesions and cancers.

Secondary smoke, or tobacco smoke in the air, can have an adverse effect on nonsmokers.

Smoking by pregnant women has been related to premature birth, spontaneous abortion, stillbirth, and neonatal death (American Cancer Society).

One of the more obvious chronic effects of smoking is that it greatly diminishes the senses of taste and smell.

Besides nicotine, tobacco smoke contains a number of potentially harmful tars, gases, and other irritants, including carbon monoxide and hydrogen cyanide. The American Cancer Society estimates that smoking two packs a day can decrease life expectancy by 8.3 years. The cancer death rate for male smokers is double that of nonsmokers. There are many more statistics just as dire. It is generally agreed that cigarette smoking is bad for health, yet tobacco is a multi-billion-dollar industry that lobbies for the continuing acceptance of its use and against any attempt at regulation.

Emergency Treatment

Smoking overdoses can be ameliorated with fresh air and lying down.

There have been rare cases of acute poisoning in which people have eaten tobacco by mistake, or have absorbed concentrated nicotine insecticides, or have consumed nicotine as part of a folk cure for worms and constipation. Such cases are serious and should have professional emergency treatment.

Long-term Treatment

There are many methods of nicotine detoxification, ranging from "cold turkey" to gradual withdrawal and using such means as hypnosis; analysis; positive reinforcement; and special, graduated filters. People have been known to throw their cigarettes away during solo ocean voyages.

The actual physical withdrawal symptoms usually go away within 1 to 3 weeks. The drug hunger may last much, much longer, in some cases an entire lifetime. Although recovery is possible, the addiction itself remains strong, and abstinent tobacco users are very vulnerable to recidivism—falling back into abuse of the drug.

METHYLPHENIDATE HYDROCHLORIDE

Chemical name: a-phenyl-2-piperidine acetic acid

Category: Schedule II

Product name: Ritalin®

Street names: West Coast, pellets

Description: White, odorless, fine crystalline powder, solutions of which are acid to litmus. Freely soluble in water.

Means of ingestion: Swallowed in tablets or sustained release tablets.

General Information

Ritalin® is similar in effect to amphetamines but chemically different and thought by some to have fewer dangerous side effects. It is used for all the principal indications for amphetamines. Its most general use, however, is in the treatment of childhood hyperkinesis. When used on children with short attention spans, emotional instability, or moderate to severe hyperactivity, it seems to have a paradoxical nonstimulant effect. No one is sure just how this drug acts. The children appear to be calmer and frequently do better in school. These children report feeling "changed" but not sedated. An adult physician who had been a medicated hyperkinetic child described the effect as: "When you're hyper it's as though all your receptor channels are going at once. The medication cuts down on the input so you can concentrate on only a few things at a time." This use is highly controversial, and there is an ongoing debate among physicians and researchers about whether basic behavior patterns are altered by Ritalin® — or, for that matter by other stimulants used for this indication. It is usually used in conjunction with counseling, psychotherapy, and other behavior-modifying treatment.

In recreational misuse, the effects are similar to those of amphetamines. Abuse is reported to be widespread.

Dangers

The dangers from Ritalin® are similar to those from amphetamines. One unique problem occurs when it is abused by injection. Ritalin® pills contain talcum as a filler and binding agent. The talc is an insoluble crystal that irritates and can cause abscesses when it is injected subcutaneously. When injected intravenously, the crystals of talc can become imbedded in lung capillaries and may cause pulmonary abscesses and fibrosis. In some cases, this condition has necessitated the removal of a lung.

Emergency Treatment

Similar to that for amphetamines.

Long-term Treatment

Similar to that for amphetamines.

MISCELLANEOUS STIMULANTS

Besides the stimulants that we have discussed individually and in depth, there are a couple of other substances that are loosely related to amphetamine and appear in the ranks of abused drugs on occasion.

Prescription Anorexiants

Phenmetrazine (Preludin®) and pemoline (Cylert®) also are similar to the amphetamines. Used in short-term weight loss as an appetite suppressant. Once more, the abuse is similar to that of amphetamine as is treatment. There are a number of other nonamphetamine anorexics (weight-reduction agents) on the market as prescription drugs. These include Bontril®, Fastin® and Ionamin®, all containing phentermine, and Tenuate®, which contains diethylpropion. Once more, these drugs resemble amphetamines and similar treatment rules would apply to their abuse.

Over-the-Counter Anorexiants

These preparations are similar in composition to the look-alike stimulants discussed earlier. They contain such nonscheduled substances as ephedrine, phenolpropanolamine, and caffeine. One major difference from the look-alike stimulants, however, is that these over-the-counter preparations are made in time-release pills and capsules. With only small amounts of the drugs being released at a time, the desired recreational effects are reduced to a point where they are rarely abused.

Psychedelics/Psychotomimetics/
Hallucinogenics

HISTORICAL PERSPECTIVE

Although they were not labeled as such until recently, psychedelic drugs have been with us for a long time. The use of cannabis, for example, is at least as old as the use of opium in the Middle East. All parts of the plant — seeds, leaves, and resin — were used medicinally, ceremonially, and recreationally before the dawn of recorded history.

Progenitors of the drugs we now call psychedelic were prominently involved in early religious practices in both the Eastern and Western hemispheres. Anthropologists and ethnobotanists have studied many ancient rituals, searching for clues to the relationship between mystical religion and substances that bring about changes in consciousness.

The "rites of spring" practiced by Classical and pre-Classical Greek mystery religions appear to have involved such substances. Ethnopharmacologists who have studied accounts of the "elysian mysteries" cite such a link. In the celebration of these mysteries, thousands of pilgrims would travel to the Greek city of Elusius to witness the rebirth of Persephone, the goddess of spring, who spends each winter in the underworld. They gathered at a temple that housed the entrance through which she returned to our world. These pilgrims were given a concoction of wine, herbs, and according to the scientists, ergotomine, in order to gain a direct perception of the goddess. Ergotomine is a psychoactive mold that grows on rye grain. It later became a prime ingredient in LSD.

Consciousness-affecting substances also played an important role in medicine. In Ancient Greece, the practice of medicine was passed down by oral tradition from master to disciple. The disciples were referred to as "sons of Aesculapius," the mythical father of medicine. Hippocrates, for example, was the fifty-seventh son, meaning that he was fifty-seventh in the line of masters from the founder.

These physicians practiced at aesklepions — healing communities not unlike modern European sanitoriums, where the sick came to be treated. The patients were given trance- and vision-producing concoctions, and their treatment was based on the visions they had.

Although cannabis and other mind-altering substances continued to be used ritually and medicinally in the Near East, India, and the Far East, the use of these drugs was lost to European science during the Middle Ages. When natural ingestion of such substances occurred by accident, such as in the ergotomine poisonings in France, the results were seen as cases of demonic possession. Contamination of bread by ergotomine, a rye grain precursor of LSD, caused villagers who ate the bread to exhibit psychotomimetic behavior.

Inhabitants of the Western Hemisphere made much use of conscious-ness-affecting substances. Although many practices went underground with the coming of European conquest and colonization, it was to native American psychedelics that western scientists first turned their attention after a long hiatus. In the 19th and 20th centuries, these scientists began to "rediscover" psychedelic drug use in primitive cultures and to experi-ment with these substances themselves.

One of the first drugs that they turned to was the button of the peyote cactus. Peyote had been used ceremonially since ancient times by Indians in Northern Mexico and what became the American Southwest. Neither the Spanish Inquisition nor a succession of American governments were able to eradicate its use as a stimulant, general medicine, and ceremonial psychedelic. Its use had in fact spread throughout Southwestern tribes in the mid-19th century as an antidote to the despair caused by the white man's eclipse and eradication of their culture.

In attempting to end its use, churches and government agencies charac-terized peyote as causing a variety of gruesome activities, none of which appear to have had any foundation in fact. Anthropologists became in-trigued by the peyote ceremony and some actually took part in it. These intrepid few, however, discovered that there were certain negative costs to the experience. These included nausea and repeated vomiting, as well as a residual bitter taste that none would ever forget. The Indian users con-sidered the nausea and vomiting to be part of an intrinsic cleansing pro-cess and accepted them, but the anthropologists were less than willing to tolerate these side effects.

In 1856, however, mescaline, the active ingredient of peyote, was iso-lated and named for the Mescalero Apaches of Northern Mexico. By the turn of the century, mescaline became available for research. Soon there-after, its structural relationship to the adrenal hormone epinephrine, which occurs naturally in the human brain, was recognized.

Sigmund Freud, William James, Havelock Ellis, and other experi-menters wrote about the drug. Their writing stimulated scholarly as well as popular interest. Pharmacologists began to explore mescaline and other substances as tools for the investigation of mental illness.

Popular interest in mescaline was further sparked by the English phi-losopher and novelist Aldous Huxley and the French artist Henri Mi-cheaux. Both men wrote directly of their experiences with the drug in terms the general public could understand. Other drugs may cause physical symptoms and effects such as euphoria, stimulation and feelings of well-being, but mescaline caused changes in the mind itself. At a time when the psychological theories of Sigmund Freud and Carl G. Jung were coming into vogue with their tantalizing glimpses of libido and mass unconscious, mescaline provided a doorway into other perceptions. In a few years, a discovery in Switzerland blew that doorway wide open.

Lysergic acid diethylamide (LSD) was first synthesized in 1938, but it was not until 1943 that the drug's profound psychological effects were first discovered. In that year, shortly after Enrico Fermi initiated the earth's first manmade nuclear chain reaction for the Manhattan Project, Dr. Albert Hofmann first developed LSD-25 for Sandoz Pharmaceuticals in Bazel, Switzerland. He accidentally ingested some of the compound and experienced visual alteration and difficulty riding home on his bicycle.

In 1938, he had been looking for an analeptic (restorative) with stimulant properties similar to those of nikethamide. Instead of discovering a new analeptic, he had, after a five-year gestation, given birth to the most controversial chemical compound of the 20th century.

Over the next two decades, LSD-25 underwent a social and medical evolution characterized by shifting professional and lay models of the drug's function.

The first of these models was the *psychotomimetic*, the psychiatric-pharmacological model. This treated the drug experience as a form of psychosis. The psychotomimetic paradigm was followed, though not necessarily superseded, by the *hallucinogenic* model, which treated LSD as a tool for studying the mechanisms of perception, and the *therapeutic model*, which represented rather an about-face from characterization as psychosis-producing. Finally, there came the *psychedelic* model, which was that under proper conditions the LSD experience would be one of enlightening and productive consciousness expansion.

With the psychedelic model, LSD began to take on a religious-mystical cast that it shared with other drugs, such as peyote and mescaline, that produced similar effects. The religious-mystical nature of LSD and other psychedelic drugs became the preoccupation of several studies of the compounds. The most notable of these was conducted at Harvard University by a group of psychologists headed by Timothy Leary and including Richard Alpert and Ralph Metzner. Under their management, creative people including artists, writers, and musicians underwent the "psychedelic experience." They proceeded to write of their experiences in books and articles and to discuss them on radio and television.

At this same time, interest in other substances was aroused. Psilocybin mushrooms had been used in Mexico for over a thousand years before the time of Columbus. This use was suppressed by the Spanish Inquisition

and their very existence came to be considered a myth. Shamanistic use
of psilocybin had continued underground, however, and was "rediscovered" in the mid-1950s.

The intoxicating qualities of nutmeg and mace were well known to
ornithologists, but the side effects limited their use among humans. Nutmeg and sassafras provided the basis along with amphetamine for a whole
class of drugs that had psychedelic properties and structure similar to
mescaline. These were the methoxelated amphetamines, many of which
had been first synthesized in Germany prior to World War I. These include the "alphabet soup" psychedelics, DOM (STP), MDA, MMDA,
MDM, and number over a thousand different but related chemical substances.

Closely related to LSD were the seeds of the morning glory and Hawaiian woodrose vines. Referred to in the street as "poor man's acid,"
these could be found growing in gardens throughout the western world.

While fewer than a dozen psychedelic plants were known in the Eastern Hemisphere, over ninety species were known and used in the Western
Hemisphere. This does not count synthesized compounds. Besides the
substances we have already named there are the harmala alkaloids, found
in the seeds of the Near Eastern shrub *Peganum harmala* (Syrian rue) and
in the bark of a variety of vines from the South American Amazon Basin;
ibogaine, which comes to us from the root of the West African plant
Tabernanthe iboga; DMT or N,N-dimethyltryptamine from South America; muscimole from the *Amanita muscaria* mushroom; and a group
called the anticholinergic deliriants that includes deadly nightshade, mandrake, black henbane, jimson weed, and over twenty other species of
henbane and datura. Finally, there are the dissociative anesthetics – phencyclidine, ketamine, and their analogues. Doubtless there are many other
consciousness-effective substances in our world as well, but these are the
ones that would most likely be encountered. Ethnobotanists and ethnopharmacologists maintain that with the exception of the Arctic and Ant-
arctic circles there are probably one or more species of psychedelic
growth in or near every inhabited point in the world.

During the 1960s the use of psychedelics became a national preoccupation and obsession among the young of the United States and Western
Europe. It shaped art, music, writing, and thought. Unfortunately, it also
caused a lot of problems.

It was during this proliferation that the presence of LSD-induced negative reactions became acute. During the clinically supervised stage in
LSD's sociopharmacological development, adverse reactions were rare.
Sidney Cohen, MD, one of the pioneer investigators of LSD, reported in
1960 that the incidence of psychotic reactions lasting more than 48 hours
was 0.8 per 1000 in patients. By the time the Haight-Ashbury Free Medical Clinic first opened its doors on the corner of Haight and Clayton

Streets in San Francisco on June 7, 1967, however, bad acid trips or bummers, as the psychedelic subculture called them, were frequent.

These psychedelic bad trips have become less and less frequent in recent years as psychedelic drug dosages have decreased and people in general have had a clearer knowledge of how to handle them. The bad trips, however, have been replaced by less frequent but more problematical long-term effects.

ACUTE PSYCHEDELIC TOXICITY

The acute effects of psychedelic drugs occur during the direct drug experience and are commonly called "bad trips." These aberrations can take many forms. Often an individual can knowingly take the drug and then fly into a state of anxiety as the powerful psychedelic begins to take effect. People are aware that they have taken a drug but feel that they cannot control its effects and want to be taken out of their state of intoxication *immediately*. This condition is similar to becoming self-conscious in the midst of a threatening dream but not being able to wake up from it. LSD users on a bad trip sometimes try to flee from the situation, giving rise to possible physical danger. Others may become highly paranoid and suspicious of their companions, treatment personnel, or others.

Not all bad trips are based on anxiety or loss of control, however. Some people on psychedelic drugs show decided changes in cognition and demonstrate poor judgment. They may have the feeling that they can fly and may jump out a window. Some users are reported to have walked into the sea, feeling that they were "part of the universe." Such physical mishaps were described within the psychedelic subculture as "being God but tripping over the furniture."

These problems have been especially evident with the dissociative drug phencyclidine (PCP). Here the body and mind are actually blocked from each other, and victims react to a variety of input distortions that may have no bearing at all on what is going on around them.

Susceptibility to bad trips is not necessarily dose related, but it does depend on the experience, maturity, and personality of the user, as well as upon the external environment in which the trip takes place. Sometimes the individual will complain of unpleasant symptoms while intoxicated and later speak in glowing terms of the experience. Negative psychological set and environmental setting were the biggest contributing factors to bad LSD trips in the 1960s.

A parallel to psychedelic bad trips can be seen in the multicultural annals of mystical religion, which describe a similarity of phenomena encountered in deep meditation and yogically altered states of consciousness. These phenomena, bearing such names as "Guardians of the Gate," or "Dwellers on the Threshold," are personified in Eastern iconography as semihuman monsters of ferocious mien and demeanor who literally guard the entrance to heaven (nirvana) and frighten away the unprepared. Much care is taken in mystical initiatory procedures to prepare initiates for dealing with these forces.

Treatment of Acute Toxicity

Most psychedelic-induced acute toxicity is best treated in a supportive, nonpharmacological fashion through the restoration of a positive, non-threatening environment. Techniques using these procedures were developed originally within the psychedelic community and used by free clinics and community-based programs. Facilities such as those occupied by the Haight-Ashbury Free Medical Clinic sprang up in the 1960s and early 1970s. These residential settings with little to mark them as "medical," with quiet space set aside for drug crises, and with casually dressed staff dedicated to a nonjudgmental attitude, were admirably suited for treating bad trips.

Most acute adverse reactions can be "talked down." Medication or hospitalization is seldom necessary.

Maintaining a relaxed, conversational tone can assist in putting the individual at ease. Quick movements should be avoided. Staff should make patients comfortable, without impeding their freedom of movement. They should be allowed to walk around, stand, lie down, or smoke if they wish. At times such physical movement and activity can be enough to break the anxiety reaction. Patients should be gently persuaded away from any activity that seems to be adding to their agitation. Getting the bad-tripper's mind off the frightening elements of the trip and onto positive elements is the key to the talk-down.

An understanding of the phases generally experienced in a psychedelic trip can be most helpful in treating acute reactions. After orally ingesting an average dose of 100 to 250 micrograms of LSD, or effective doses of other psychedelic drugs, the user usually experiences sympathomimetic responses that include elevated heart rate and stimulated respiration and pulse. Adverse reactions in this phase are primarily anxiety reactions. These tend to occur in novices and generally are managed by reassurances that the observed experiences are normal and expected effects of psychedelics. Reassurance is usually sufficient to change and defuse a potentially frightening situation.

From the first to the sixth hour, with LSD, visual imagery becomes vivid and may take on frightening content. The patient may forget having taken the drug or — given acute time distortion — may believe this retinal circus will go on forever. Such fears can be dispelled by reminding the individual that these effects *are* drug induced, by suggesting alternative images, and by distracting the individual from images that are frightening.

In the later stages thoughts, insights, and philosophical ideas may predominate. Adverse experiences here are most frequently due to unpleasant recurring thoughts or feelings which can become overwhelming in their impact. The therapist can be most effective by being supportive and by suggesting new trains of thought.

The therapist's attitude toward the situation is very important. Empathy and self-confidence are essential. Anxiety or fear in the therapist may be amplified in the patient's perceptions. Physical contact with the individual is often reassuring but can be misinterpreted. Often the therapist must rely on intuition and a clear reading of the patient.

In extreme cases — if the therapist cannot establish any contact with the patient, if the talk-down has failed, or if anxiety continues to override this treatment — medication may be necessary. If so, oral administration of a sedative, such as 25 mg of chlordiazepoxide (Librium®) or 10 mg of diazepam (Valium®), can have an important pharmacological and reassurance effect.

During the second and third phases, a toxic psychosis or major break with reality may occur, in which one can no longer communicate with the patient. If the individual begins acting in such a way as to be an immediate danger, antipsychotic drugs may be employed. Only if the individual refuses oral medication and is out of behavioral control do we suggest administering antipsychotics by injection. Haldol®, 2 to 4 mg given intramuscularly followed by evaluation and readministration as needed, is the current drug of choice. Any use of medication, however, should only be undertaken by qualified personnel. If antipsychotic drugs are required, hospitalization is usually indicated. However, we have found that most bad acid trips can be handled on an outpatient basis with the medication being the talk-down.

As soon as rapport and verbal contact are established, further medication is generally not necessary. Occasionally an individual fails to respond to the above regimen and must be referred to an inpatient psychiatric facility. Such a decision must be weighed carefully, however, for transfer to a hospital may exacerbate the patient's bad trip. Hospitalization should be used only as a last resort.

In general, the treatment procedures described are geared to LSD, which is the most powerful psychedelic on a per-dose basis and also in terms of intensity of effects. The bad trips caused by other psychedelics vary in duration, as do their drug effects in general. All specific drug information should be consulted for variations.

Phencyclidine presents its own symptomatology and procedures for handling both acute and chronic toxicity. Although these general guidelines may be helpful, be sure to consult the section on phencyclidine when dealing with victims of that drug, ketamine, and other PCP analogues.

CHRONIC PSYCHEDELIC TOXICITY

Chronic toxicity presents situations wherein a condition that may be attributable to the ingestion of a toxic substance occurs or continues long after the metabolization of that substance. In the use of psychedelics, four recognized chronic reactions have been reported:

1. Prolonged psychotic reactions
2. Depression sufficiently severe to be life threatening
3. Flashbacks
4. Exacerbation of preexisting psychiatric illness

Some people who have taken many psychedelic trips, especially those who have had acute adverse reactions, develop what appears to be a serious long-term personality disruption. These prolonged psychotic reactions have similarities to schizophrenic reactions and appear to occur most often in people with preexisting psychological difficulties — primarily prepsychotic or psychotic personalities. Psychedelic-induced personality disorders can be quite severe and prolonged. Appropriate treatment often requires antipsychotic medication and residential care in a mental health facility, followed by long-term outpatient counseling. In certain cases, psychedelic-induced chronic psychological problems lead to complicated patterns of polydrug abuse that require additional treatment approaches.

By far the most ubiquitous chronic reaction to LSD and the stronger psychedelics is the flashback. Flashbacks are transient spontaneous occurrences of some aspect of the drug effect occurring after a period of normalcy following the original intoxication. This period of normalcy distinguishes flashbacks from prolonged psychotic reactions.

The drug-related quality of the experience is frequently stressed. Flashbacks may occur after a single ingestion of a psychedelic, but more commonly they occur after multiple psychedelic drug ingestions. The flashback experience has also been reported following the use of marijuana. Flashbacks have been reported to occur during times of stress, relaxation, or everyday activities; during intoxication by alcohol, barbiturates, or marijuana; and during ingestion of antihistamines and accompanying viral infections.

Flashbacks are a symptom, not a specific disease entity. They may well have multiple etiologies, and many instances that have been identified as flashbacks might have occurred had the individual never ingested a psychedelic drug. Although some investigators have postulated that these occurrences may be due to a residue of drug that is released into the system at a later time, there is no direct evidence of psychedelic retention or prolonged storage. Health professionals whose training is oriented toward psychology usually evoke psychological explanations for flashbacks, while those who are physiologically oriented attempt to explain the phenomenon in physical terms.

Nor is there agreement about whether flashbacks in and of themselves are a good or a bad thing. Given the intensity of the states of altered consciousness encountered during a psychedelic experience, an individual may become unusually aware of natural changes in visual, perceptual, or body sensations which do not usually reach conscious awareness. Once awareness of the sensation has been noted, however, a noticed recurrence of that sensation may form the basis of a flashback. If the individual attaches a negative connotation to the experience, then anxiety and fear are produced. A circular reinforcing process can escalate the occurrence to panic proportions.

In general, chronic aftereffects of psychedelics can be worked with in a reassuring manner. Flashbacks, for example, usually fade in time. They have not been known to recur more than a year after the last psychedelic trip. Feelings of dissociation or emotional flattening out also fade with time. Clients with such long-term problems should be guided toward life-reinforcing activities that involve positive interactions with other people. Helpful too are such self-reintegrating activities as running, aerobic exercise, artistic endeavor, yoga, and meditation. All counseling should include frequent reminders that the problem is transitory. The person's case is not unusual, and the prognosis is always positive (Smith & Seymour, 1985).

CANNABIS SATIVA/CANNABIS INDICA

Chemical name: Delta-9, tetrahydrocannabinol

Category: Schedule II

Product names: None

Street names: Marijuana, Mary Jane, jay, smoke, reefer, hashish, pot, dope, ganja, gange, hemp, weed, dagga, sinsemilla, charas, etc.

Description: Vegetable matter, either leaves or long leafy buds ranging in color from bright green to dark brown or golden. May smell "skunky" or like perfume. Often sold as buds or with clumps of leaves still on portions of stalk. Rarely, it is seeded and semipulverized, but this form is considered not very potent. Sinsemilla grown in the United States is both highly potent and expensive. It usually appears as very long, large buds. Another highly prized form of marijuana is the Tai stick. Marijuana is manicured for seeds and wound around a short piece of split bamboo.

The usual sales unit of marijuana is the "lid," which is usually about an ounce in weight and comes in sandwich "baggies." In urban areas, it is also sold by the "joint," or prerolled marijuana cigarette. Marijuana may also be retailed by the half-ounce, gram, or — going the other way — by the pound or kilo (kilogram or 2.2 pounds). When most marijuana was imported from Mexico, it came in pressed 1-kilogram bricks.

Hashish is the highly potent resin of the cannabis plant. It is extracted from the marijuana in a variety of colorful ways and sold by the gram, ounce, or pound. The substance varies in color from yellow through chocolate brown to green and greenish black. It ranges in consistency from powdery to Mexican chocolate-like to hard and tarlike. The resin is usually packed into cakes, lumps, or balls.

Cannabis resin can also be extracted with solvents and concentrated into a thick, oily liquid called hash oil.

Means of ingestion: Marijuana, hashish, and hash oil can be smoked, eaten, infused into a tea, or swallowed in pills or capsules but not insufflated or injected.

General Information

Cannabis (*indica* or *sativa*) has been used medicinally and recreationally for over 2000 years. Its use is widespread through a number of cultures and it has been smoked in cigarettes (joints or spliffs), pipes, chillums, and bongs to name only a few. It has been eaten by itself or cooked into just about anything from chocolate brownies to spaghetti sauce. In many cultures, marijuana is infused into a tea and used for childhood gastrointestinal distress. As hemp, cannabis is widely cultivated for the making of rope.

Like wine, marijuana has different tastes and potencies depending on where and how it is grown and cured. Until recently, American strains were considered inferior to the highly potent marijuana and hashish of Nepal, Tibet, Afghanistan, and Thailand. In the past decade, however, much covert technology has been applied to American sinsemilla. It may now be the equal of or superior to many indica strains. Indica is the cannabis classification grown in the Eastern Hemisphere, while sativa is that grown in the Western Hemisphere.

Cannabis enjoys a world-wide folklore, as evidenced by the variety of names. More research has been done on marijuana than on any other psychoactive substance with the exception of alcohol and tobacco. Findings are often contradictory, however, and many aspects of marijuana, including its long-term effects, remain obscure. Research is further complicated by the presence of highly emotional reactions to the drug. Its protagonists claim that it is not harmful at all, while its antagonists produce long lists of permanent adverse effects.

Research on possible medical uses continues. This research involves both marijuana itself and an active ingredient, delta-9 tetrahydrocannabinol, which has been synthesized and is being tested in pill form. Possible uses include the treatment of glaucoma, asthma, epilepsy, and nausea related to cancer chemotherapy.

The onset of effects when cannabis is smoked is very rapid, and the effects usually last for several hours. When it is eaten, the onset is slower but the effects may be of longer duration and more profound. The effects of marijuana and hashish range from euphoria to dysphoria, depending on potency, setting, orientation, expectation, and state of mind.

Dangers

A committee of the Institute of Medicine recently concluded: "The scientific evidence published to date indicates that marijuana has a broad range of psychological and biological effects, some of which, at least under certain conditions, are harmful to human health. Unfortunately, the available information does not tell us how serious these risks may be" (Relman, 1982).

Daily heavy inhalation of marijuana smoke, which contains tars and other substances similar to those found in tobacco, can produce bronchial irritation and may lead to long-term pulmonary damage (Smith & Seymour, 1981). There is no hard evidence, however, for the hypothesis that marijuana is 20 times more carcinogenic than tobacco. Excessive marijuana use by very young people may have some responsibility for a decreased desire to work or compete, but these problems involve about 3% of marijuana users. We do, however, view the compulsive and chronic use of marijuana, like chronic alcohol use, especially by the very young, as counterproductive and unhealthy, both to the culture and to the individual.

There is still very much speculation and controversy over marijuana's effects on the nervous system and behavior, the cardiovascular and respiratory systems, the respiratory system and chromosomes, and the immune system. For years, the polarizing emotionalism of promarijuana and antimarijuana forces has clouded the judgment of both factions. The former have hypothesized claims on the basis of inadequate and often contradictory data while the latter often attempt to ignore even the clinically verifiable dangers.

Despite the differences over long-term effects, there is some agreement on the short-term, or acute, problems. These occur either while the active ingredients are still in the body or shortly thereafter and can include nausea, anxiety, paranoia and disorientation. There are also a variety of minor symptoms not normally considered adverse reactions, including reddening of the eyes, dryness of the mouth, sudden hunger, and sedation. The reaction to these by the user ranges from annoyance to welcome indications that one is high.

Some of the more unpleasant consequences of use are disorientation, confused states, short-term memory loss, and a variety of perceptual moods and conceptual alterations. These effects are especially likely to be perceived as unpleasant if they produce concern or fear rather than the emotional state desired. Anxiety reactions and paranoid toxic psychosis may be serious enough to lead the user to seek professional help.

There are some clear dangers involved in marijuana use. The drug additive effect, for example, especially between marijuana and alcohol, can render one dysfunctional and physically ill. Overindulgence in marijuana can cause nausea, dizziness, and unpleasant "drugged" feelings, similar to being drunk and sick on alcohol. The evidence is clear that one should not drive or run any kind of machinery while high on marijuana. It is also becoming clear that metabolites of cannabis that are fat soluable remain in the body for a long time. There does not seem to be a prolonged psychoactive effect or cumulative effect from this retention, however.

Victims of addictive disease who are in recovery and abstention should totally avoid the use of cannabis. It can act as a trigger to restimulate drug hunger for one's drug of choice and could bring about readdiction. This is true of any psychoactive drug. This does not mean that use of marijuana will lead to use of narcotics and other drugs (Seymour & Smith, 1983).

A final danger comes not from cannabis itself but from attempts to stop its use. This is the hypothetical danger from the smoking of cannabis contaminated from paraquat or other herbicides. A study on this subject carried out by the Centers for Disease Control ended in complete confusion but did bring a halt to spraying of marijuana crops in 1978. However, resumption of such spraying is still considered a viable alternative by various domestic and international agencies. Such a program could further jeopardize the lives and health of all concerned (Smith & Seymour, 1979; Seymour, 1982).

Emergency Treatment

Panic reactions are usually short term and can be easily managed with reassurance. Advanced paranoid reactions can be reversed by standard psychedelic talk-down techniques. In extreme cases, hospitalization and medication with minor tranquilizers may be necessary.

Long-term Treatment

Compulsive use may be stopped through total support of abstinence on the order of Alcoholics Anonymous or Narcotics Anonymous programs or through supportive counseling and self-help. Acupuncture, biofeedback, and meditation as well as regular aerobic exercise have been effective.

Long-term problems or situations in which marijuana is being used to self-medicate underlying psychological problems call for appropriate counseling by health professionals.

All currently recognized adverse effects are fully reversible through sustained abstinence.

DOB

Chemical name: 4-bromo-2, t-dimethoxy-amphetamine

Category: Unscheduled at this time

Product names: None

Street names: Golden Eagles, tiles

Description: A drug of deception for LSD, DOB is most often sold as a liquid or powder, or on a one-centimeter absorbent paper "blot" with a green bird on a yellow or white background (Golden Eagle), or with a black and white geometrical pattern (tile) (Bowen, 1983).

Means of ingestion: Eaten

General Information

DOB is an analogue or varient of 4-methyl-2,5-dimethoxyamphetamine, otherwise known as STP or DOM. In this analogue, the four methyl atoms have been exchanged for four bromo atoms. Otherwise, the valence or chemical balance of the molecule remains the same. An analogue is just such a minor change in the molecular structure of a drug in which the basic structure, and effects, remain similar. Both drugs have hallucinogenic properties similar to those of LSD. DOB is also one of the "methoxylated amphetamines," also discussed under that general heading, and has both psychedelic and stimulant effects.

Among the methoxylated amphetamines, there is a great difference in dosage and effect. MDA, for example, has a minimum "threshold" (effective) dosage of 100 to 150 mg and a duration of 8 to 12 hours. STP or DOM, which DOB most closely resembles, has an effective threshold of 5 mg and a duration of 16 to more than 24 hours.

DOB is even more potent than STP. Because of its potency, DOB has been seen as a drug of deception. It is often sold as LSD-25 because its extremely low threshold dosage makes it possible for DOB to be dropped on small blotter sheets. In this form, it can pass for blotter acid. Users expecting a usual-duration acid trip, however, can be unpleasantly surprised — and seriously alarmed — by the exceptional duration and intensity of DOB.

The usual dose of DOB is 1 to 5 mg. The drug takes effect about an hour after ingestion, and the effects last from 12 to 24 hours. Physical symptoms include an increase in pulse rate, increased systolic blood pressure, and dilation of the eye pupils. The bromine in DOB seems to delay the metabolic breakdown and elimination of this drug from the system. There is evidence that tolerance to DOB develops (Delliou, 1980).

Dangers

DOB is a very dangerous drug. As a drug of deception, DOB is a prime example of the risks taken by street users when they do not know what they are getting and what it does. Overdoses can cause psychiatric dissociation, panic, violent behavior, and death. These overdose symptoms are similar to those of other powerful stimulants.

What is especially dangerous with this particular stimulant, however, is that it can cause spasms in arm and leg blood vessels, which can and have resulted in cellular necrosis, or tissue death, and subsequent amputation. Most stimulants have some vasoconstrictive (blood vessel-tightening) effects. They shrink blood vessels. But with DOB, this effect is most pronounced.

Amphetamines have been linked to cellular necrosis in arms, legs, toes, and fingers. Localized vasospasm — complete obstruction of arteries — has resulted from hypodermic injection of phenmetrazine hydrochloride (Preludin®), as has cerebral vasculitis (inflammation of the blood vessels in the brain).

One case report of a death associated with DOB suggested cerebral edema — flooding of the brain with fluid — and seizures as the cause of death. These probably were caused by vasospasm (Wineck, 1981).

What DOB actually does is to cause diffuse vascular spasm. These spasms result in the partial or complete closing of arteries in the arms and legs. The action is not unlike what happens when a tourniquet is applied to stop arterial bleeding. The flow of blood to the extremities is totally obstructed. If this goes on for any appreciable length of time, gangrene sets in, the limbs that are affected begin to rot, and amputation becomes necessary to save the person's life.

According to the *Journal of the American Medical Association*, no amphetamine other than DOB is known to cause this extent of diffuse vascular spasm. Amphetamines do, however, produce other adverse blood-supply effects in the arms and legs, in part by releasing the neurotransmitter norepinephrine from the central nervous system. The release of norepinephrine is part of the receptor-site mechanism typical of all stimulants (Bowen, 1983).

Two overdose cases have been intensively reported, one in northern California and one in the San Diego area of Southern California. One patient knew she was taking DOB, while the second thought he was taking "LSD-25 from Mexico." The "LSD" was tested and proved to be pure DOB. Both patients had been in good health previous to taking the drug. The male patient responded to treatment with tolazoline hydrochloride (Prisculine®), a potent vasodilator (blood vessel relaxant), but the female patient eventually had both legs amputated below the knees.

Symptoms of diffuse vascular spasms include progressively aggravated paresthesias (ghost sensations) in the arms and legs, coldness of the extremities, and finally severe localized pain in the extremities. The skin of the hands, wrists, and/or feet and ankles can become bluish and mottled. The pulse may be imperceptible. Lameness and muscular pain may precede other symptoms, and localized paralysis may follow (Citron, 1970).

Emergency Treatment

Treatment information for general bad trips and other reactions to psychedelics and stimulant overdoses can be used for these DOB reactions and are to be found in the appropriate sections of this book.

The extreme vascular distress we have described above does not occur with any other known psychedelic or stimulant drug, including the methoxylated amphetamines such as MDA and STP. If these symptoms do occur, medical help should be sought immediately. If at all possible, a sample of the drug should be analyzed and the suspicion that it may be DOB should be stated. This drug, a halogenated and methoxylated amphetamine, has now been implicated in two documented cases of diffuse arterial spasm. Undoubtedly it has caused others that have not been reported.

DOB's strong serotonin agonist properties suggest a possible mechanism of action. Treatment with the vasodilators tolazoline and sodium nitroprusside in an appropriate medical setting is effective in rapidly restoring limb circulation and relieving symptoms.

Long-term Treatment

If all goes well, the acute vascular distress will not recur once it has been reversed. One episode of this kind should be enough to discourage any further use of at least this particular drug.

As with any psychedelic, problems may arise from its use that may require prolonged psychiatric care.

LSD

Chemical name: Lysergic acid diethylamide

Category: Schedule I

Product names: None

Street names: LSD, LSD-25, acid, sandoz, space caps, sunshine, owsley white lightning, blotter acid, windowpane, etc.

Description: Typically appears as a liquid added to another agent. Dosages are minute when compared with virtually all other drugs and are measured in micrograms (μg) rather than milligrams.

Means of ingestion: LSD is usually ingested orally. A tiny measured dose can be soaked into any pill or capsule. Two popular agents in the 1960s were sugar cubes and small empty capsules ("space caps"). Doses were also mixed with orange juice, Kool-Aid or other liquids. Later, LSD was mixed into a thin gel and cut into small units (windowpane) or placed in series on pieces of paper (blotter acid).

General Information

Lysergic acid diethylamide is a synthetic psychoactive drug derived from natural ergot alkaloids that are produced by the ergot fungus growing on rye grain. LSD was first synthesized in 1938 by Dr. Albert Hofmann, a chemist for Sandoz Pharmaceuticals in Switzerland. Its effects were not discovered until 1943, however, when Dr. Hofmann accidentally ingested a minute quantity of the drug. His subjective reaction led him to realize that this was the most powerful psychoactive substance he had ever encountered. It was indeed a substance so powerful that effective dosages had to be measured in micrograms rather than milligrams.

During the 1960s and early 1970s, street dosages of several hundred micrograms were the standard. After two decades of psychological experimentation, the drug had spread into a growing youth culture as the mass media created excitement about its effects, research psychologists turned guru touted its value as a psychedelic (consciousness-expanding) drug, and underground chemists learned how to synthesize it for a mass market. Users took LSD as a means to "consciousness expansion" and "cosmic liberation." Its use became central to the counterculture that thrived in the sixties and seventies, influencing art, music, philosophy, and lifestyle as no other drug has done before or since.

The onset of effects can range from 15 minutes to an hour. The effects vary greatly depending on the individual, the situation in which LSD is taken, and the mental state of the user.

In recent years, a standard dose has been 50 to 75 micrograms, taken recreationally for its euphoric effects and intoxication rather than for consciousness expansion. There are indications, however, that a nostalgia for the sixties is prompting higher dosages.

Dangers

The dangers of LSD can be divided into acute effects and chronic aftereffects as follow. The **acute effects** occur during the acid experience and are commonly known as "bad trips." These can include anxiety, fear over loss of control, paranoia, and delusions of persecution or of grandeur. Some people on LSD show decided changes in cognition and demonstrate poor judgment. Susceptibility to bad trips is not necessarily dose related but does involve the experience, maturity, and personality of the user. Smaller doses and widespread knowledge of how to handle them have greatly decreased the clinical incidence of bad LSD trips.

There are four recognized **chronic aftereffects** to LSD use: (1) prolonged psychotic reactions, (2) severe, life-threatening depression, (3) flashbacks, and (4) exacerbation of preexisting psychiatric illness.

Taking LSD can be very dangerous for someone with a history of psychological difficulties or psychiatric illness. The prolonged psychotic reactions have similarities to schizophrenia and occur most often with prepsychotic personalities. These disturbances can be both severe and lengthy.

Flashbacks are transient, spontaneous recurrences of psychedelic drug experiences that take place after a period of normalcy. The period of normalcy is what distinguishes flashback from prolonged psychotic reactions. Subjective reactions to flashbacks can range from pleasure to terror and anxiety. Flashbacks can occur during times of stress, during relaxation, or during everyday activities; during intoxication by alcohol, barbiturates, or marijuana; and during ingestion of antihistamines or in the course of viral infections. No one is sure what causes them. They do, however, fade with time. None has been recorded more than a year after the last use of a psychedelic drug.

Despite long-standing assertions of chromosomal damage, there is no evidence that LSD is retained in the body for extended periods. Although LSD use has been connected with the perpetrators of some spectacular crimes, LSD itself does not appear to be a precipitating factor. Overdoses are not physically dangerous, nor is LSD habit- or dependency-forming. There is no evidence of tolerance development, and the nature of the drug's effect tends to preclude serial use or binging.

Emergency Treatment

Talk-downs of most acute LSD reactions can usually be accomplished without medication or hospitalization. It is important to maintain a relaxed conversational tone, to avoid quick movements, and to make the person comfortable without impeding freedom of movement. Patients should be encouraged to walk around, stand, lie down, smoke — whatever they like. This kind of activity may act to break the anxiety reaction. Gentle suggestion should be used to keep the person from making any dangerous moves. Subdued lighting and sound and restful surroundings help. It is critical to get the person's mind off what is frightening about the experience and onto more positive aspects. Physical contact can help: Intuition, empathy, and self-confidence should be the guides to action.

Long-term Treatment

Flashbacks are a rare occurrence and do not occur more than a year after the last ingestion of a psychedelic drug. An adverse reaction to a flashback can be treated by talking the patient down. Fears can be dealt with in counseling, including the reminder that such occurrences are limited in time.

Psychotic reactions, depression, and exacerbations of psychiatric illness may call for hospitalization and the use of antipsychotic medication. In these cases, long-term counseling and other treatment are often necessary (Smith & Seymour, 1985).

MESCALINE/PEYOTE

Chemical name: 3,4,5-trimethoxyphenylethylamine

Category: Schedule I

Product names: None

Street names: Mescal, mescalito, buttons, cactus, crystals, peyotl, hikuri

Description: Mescaline appears as long, needlelike white crystals. Peyote is the button-shaped buds of the peyote cactus. They are light green to dark brown, depending on the time since they were harvested and the way in which they are preserved. These buttons have an indented patch of white filaments or fuzz at their center.

Means of ingestion: Mescaline can be taken in capsules or dissolved in water or other liquids and swallowed. Peyote is either chewed or steeped in a tea. Usually, the white filaments are removed before they are ingested. These hairs are popularly thought to be poisonous, containing strychnine but are actually just cellulose. They are indigestible but not poisonous.

General Information

Mescaline, or 3,4,5-trimethoxyphenylethylamine, is a phenylalkylamine derived from the peyote or peyotl cactus, which grows in northern South America, Mexico, and the southwestern United States, and from the San Pedro cactus of Peru (Grinspoon & Bakalar, 1979). Mescaline and peyote have similar psychedelic effects, although the greater hallucinogenic powers of peyote lead us to believe that the plant probably contains other psychoactive elements besides mescaline.

Mescaline was first isolated from peyote at the turn of the century. Until the synthesis of LSD and the rediscovery of psilocybin in the 1950s, mescaline served as an introduction to altered states of consciousness for many writers and other creative people in the Western world. Notable among these were the British philosopher and writer Aldous Huxley and the French artist Henri Micheaux, who wrote about their experiences with the drug (Huxley, 1954; Micheaux, 1956).

Mescaline has about one three-hundredths the potency of LSD, but the effects are similar and the experience lasts about the same length of time. Both mescaline and peyote are reported to be more sensual and perceptual in their action than is LSD, with less change in thought, mood, and sense of self.

Peyote, the parent drug, has been used by American Indians since ancient times as a stimulant, general medicine, and ceremonial psychedelic. Spanish conquerors carrying the Spanish Inquisition to the New World, and a succession of Mexican and American governments, have tried to stamp out the use of peyote. This use spread throughout the southwestern United States during the 19th century, in part as an antidote to Indian despair over the spread of European immigrants westward.

Although peyote is generally an illegal drug and on Schedule I along with mescaline, its ritual use by the 200,000 or more Native American congregants of the Native American Church is protected by the United States government, having been declared legal after years of court battles. As a consequence of this legality, however, the cactus has now been overharvested to the point where it may become an endangered plant species.

Peyote has played an important and ongoing role in Native American ritual and shamanism. This is indicated by its frequent discussion in the "Don Juan" works by Carlos Castaneda, and in many anthropological monographs. During the westward migration of whites, use of the psychedelic cactus swept through Indian populations who were in despair over the loss of tribal lands, the slaughter of game and their people, and the eradication of their way of life. Peyote ritual became part of, and later replaced, the Ghost Dance as a means of reaffirming spiritual values for the southwestern tribes.

Fearing the influence of peyote on Indians, government agencies and churches mounted a "reefer madness"-type attempt to discredit the drug and its use. They charged that peyote makes Indians crazy and violent, that Indians have hacked helpless victims to death, and that Indian women under its influence have ripped off their clothes in sexual frenzies (Weil & Rosen, 1983). In actuality, physical activity during intoxication is usually limited to the prescribed ritual behavior. Unlike LSD, peyote and mescaline leave one's sense of self relatively intact, while giving one intense and vivid visual effects of a colorful, complicated and often geometrical nature. This imagery is often echoed in the geometrical and colorful designs on artifacts and handcrafts from areas where peyote has been used.

Dangers

Peyote and mescaline can produce anxiety, disorientation, and dissociation with reality, especially at high dosages or as a result of fear of the drugs' effects. These feelings usually pass or can be talked through. Prolonged psychotic reactions are rare. Peyote has a nauseating, bitter taste that is not soon forgotten. It may be hard to swallow. Both peyote and mescaline often cause vomiting. Ritual users consider this to be part of the drugs' purifying effect and accept vomiting as intrinsic to the experience. Removal of the white fibers in peyote seems to have no relation to this side effect.

Other drugs, such as LSD and PCP, may be sold as mescaline, which is becoming rare and harder to find as the supply of peyote cactus diminishes (Anderson, 1980).

Emergency Treatment

A talk-down procedure similar to that used for LSD bad trips is effective for acute adverse reactions. Talk-downs should be supportive and comforting. External stimulation should be limited, and the individual should lie down and relax.

Indians have used chanting and ritualization to counter adverse effects. Tobacco smoke blown into the user's face seems to be effective, though we do not know why.

The effects of both mescaline and peyote rarely last more than 12 hours.

Long-term Treatment

Although such cases are rare, these drugs could produce the same longer-term reactions that are seen with other psychedelic drugs. These could include flashback and the triggering of latent psychological problems. Such long-term problems would be dealt with similarly to those resulting from the use of LSD and other psychedelics.

METHOXYLATED AMPHETAMINES

Chemical names: Methylenedioxyamphetamine, etc.

Category: The drugs in this class that are currently scheduled are in Schedule I.

Product names: MDA, MMDA, DOM (STP), DOET, TMA, DMMA, MDMA, MDM, etc.

Street names: The love drug, psychedelic speed, ADM, adam, XTC, ecstasy, etc.

Description: Marketed in either capsule, tablet or powder form. Powder is often creamy or off-white in color.

Means of ingestion: Usually swallowed.

General Information

Methoxylated amphetamines or psychotomimetic amphetamines are a family of drugs that represent an amphetamine subgroup and collectively exhibit the effects of both stimulants and psychedelics. The members of this family are amphetamine analogues of the psychedelic drug mescaline (methoxylated phenylethylamine). This group contains more than a thousand different but related chemical substances. Only a few have been tested on humans — in the dozens — and only a few hundred have been tested on animals. The more well-known are: MDA, MMDA, DOM (STP), DOET, TMA, DMA, DMMDA, and most recently, MDMA. All of these are similar in chemical structure and effect. They differ mostly in dosage and duration of effect. For example, MDA dosage is 100 to 150 mg and duration is 8 to 12 hours, while DOM (known on the street as STP) is potent at 5 mg and can last so long, ebbing and returning, that the user may think the trip will never end.

A possible exception to the above may be MDMA (methylendioxymethamphetamine), a recent addition to the family. Also known as MDM, Adam, and XTC, this drug was being used for research and as an adjunct to psychotherapy until July of 1985, when it was placed on emergency Schedule I by the DEA. Researchers who were working with this drug claim that its effects are quite different from other methoxylated amphetamines, and these differences make the drug valuable as a treatment tool. There is some street use of this drug, but it is difficult to ascertain how much because much of what appears as Adam or XTC (ecstasy) may actually be other drugs in this family, most often MDA.

MDA and its analogues are synthetic, but related to safrole. The natural substance is found in oil of sassafras and oil of camphor and is the psychoactive agent in nutmeg and mace. MDA has been on the street since 1967, when it first appeared in the Haight-Ashbury drug culture.

Although STP had a brief flare of popularity, most users were put off by its long duration of effectiveness. MDA is the drug in this family that has seen the most use over time and is therefore the one we know the most about. Users have reported the onset as a warm glow spreading through their bodies, followed by a sense of physical and mental well-being that gradually but steadily intensifies. Some have described a sense of increased coordination and an ability to do things they could not ordinarily do, such as sitting in meditation or doing yoga and related relaxation and centering activities for long periods of time. This effect may be due to the fact that MDA, unlike most stimulants, does not increase motor activity. Rather, it suppresses it.

It has been noted that chronic marijuana or tobacco smokers and coffee drinkers often lose all desire for these drugs during MDA's effective span. For clinical subjects in a 1974 research program, MDA served as an appetite depressant.

Some researchers have concluded that MDA produces feelings of esthetic delight, empathy, serenity, joy, insight, and self-awareness without perceptual changes, loss of control, or depersonalization — at the same time seeming to eliminate anxiety and defensiveness. "The user actually feels himself to be a child, and relives childhood experiences in full immediacy, while simultaneously remaining aware of his present self and present reality" (Turek et al., 1974).

MDA and MMDA showed great promise as an adjunct to psychotherapy in extensive research carried out in the late 1960s and early 1970s — most prominently by Claudio Naranjo of Chile and Alexander T. Shulgin (Naranjo, 1975; Shulgin, 1976). In the mid-1970s, with MDA's inclusion as a Schedule I drug, research on the methoxylated amphetamines came to a standstill until the advent of MDMA.

Dangers

As is true with all psychedelic drugs, effects vary with expectation and setting. MDA is not the sort of drug to be taken with alcohol and downers at wild parties. Actually no drug is, including alcohol and downers. MDA can drain energy, leaving one tired and sluggish the next day. It may affect a woman's genitourinary tract and may even activate latent infections there. Women should be aware of this danger.

It is reported to cause tension in the face and jaw muscles to the point of bruxism (involuntary teeth grinding). Nystagmus (jerky eye movement) has also been noticed. Anxiety, panic, or paranoid reactions can occur at high dosages and account for most treatment visits involving these drugs.

Naranjo warns that MDA is toxic to certain individuals. Typical toxic symptoms are skin reactions, profuse sweating, or confusion. A few of the more serious reported cases involved aphasia, and one death has been reported. This serious neurological toxicity results from elevated blood pressure and effects on the brain associated with higher doses of MDA.

Emergency Treatment

Nystagmus and jaw clenching are considered transitory effects of the drugs. Patients should be told or reminded that this is the case. Chewing gum can help relieve the jaw clenching.

Anxiety, panic, or paranoid reactions can usually be handled through talk-down and reassurance in a supportive environment. An elevated heartbeat and pulse is again symptomatic of the drug itself and not a threatening occurrence. In extreme cases, oral low dose diazepam (Valium®) is recommended.

Long-term Treatment

If a prolonged psychotic reaction occurs, antipsychotic medication such as Haldol® and hospitalization may be necessary. This usually happens only in individuals who have major underlying psychological problems prior to taking these drugs. In these rare cases, prolonged psychiatric care may be needed.

MORNING GLORY/HAWAIIAN WOODROSE

Chemical names: ergine (d-lysergic acid amide) and iso-ergine

Category: Not scheduled

Product names: Rivea corymbosa, Flying Saucers, tlitliltzin, badoh negro, Heavenly Blue, *ipomoea tuberosa*, Pearly Gates, ololiuqui, elephant creeper, *argyreia nervosa*, etc.

Street names: Morning glory seeds, Hawaiian baby woodrose, woodrose, poor man's acid

Description: Seeds of the morning glory and Hawaiian woodrose. The plants themselves are creeper vines that bear small flowers of a variety of colors. These vines appear in the wild and are grown decoratively in many parts of the world.

Means of ingestion: The seeds are eaten whole, ground and eaten, or leached with water which is then drunk.

General Information

In the 1950s, certain species of the common morning glory vines and their close relatives, the Hawaiian baby woodroses, were discovered to have psychedelic properties similar to those of LSD-25. The psychoactive principles of these plants comprise several forms of lysergic acid amides, chiefly ergine (*d*-lysergic acid amide) and iso-ergine. The potency is about 5 to 10% that of LSD. These alkaloids are referred to as "ergot alkaloids" because they are identical to the psychotropic LSD-type alkaloids found in ergot fungus. It is estimated that 100 morning glory seeds or 4 to 8 Hawaiian baby woodrose seeds are the equivalent of 100 micrograms of LSD.

Although ergot alkaloid-producing morning glories grow in many parts of the world, their ritual use as drugs was apparently confined to Mexico and Central America. The most notable ritual uses were with the Aztec divine plant ololiuqui (*Rivea corymbosa*) and the Mexican Indian drug tlitliltzin, or badoh negro, derived from *Ipomoea violacea*. These species of morning glory are cultivated in several ornamental varieties that include Heavenly Blue, Pearly Gates, and Flying Saucer.

Modern use of these plants for their psychedelic effects began in the late 1950s and peaked in the mid-1960s. In 1959, Albert Hofmann, the Swiss chemist who first synthesized LSD-25 from ergot fungus in the 1930s and discovered its properties in 1942, isolated the lysergic acid amides in ololiuqui seeds. The psychoactive potential of Hawaiian baby woodrose seeds was introduced to the public in 1965 in a scientific paper crediting these seeds with several times the potency of morning glory seeds.

Ingestion of these seeds was never extensive. They served as a poor substitute for LSD when the latter was scarce and more desirable psychedelics were unavailable (Grinspoon & Bakalar, 1979; Hylin & Watson, 1965; Shawcross, 1983).

Dangers

The two primary drawbacks of these substances as drugs of recreation were their lack of potency coupled with rapidly developing tolerance. Many users decided that although they had some psychedelic effect at first, this may have been a placebo effect.

Another discouraging factor was the intense abdominal cramping that seems to have inevitably accompanied a psychedelic dose. The cramping, nausea, and frequent diarrhea that accompany the use of these seeds gave rise to a street belief that the seeds either contained strychnine naturally or were coated with poison by seed companies to discourage ingestion. The general feeling among users was that the trip was not worth the side effects.

Given the low potency of the seeds, physical distress is much more probable than psychological disruption. There is a possibility of panic reactions and other psychedelic bad-trip symptoms, however, and especially in users who are unfamiliar with psychedelic effects. High doses can be dangerous and should be strictly avoided.

Emergency Treatment

Nausea and abdominal distress appear to be intrinsic. For adverse reactions, a talk-down similar to that used for LSD bad trips is effective. Personnel should be supportive and comforting and should remind the user that the overall effects usually last less than 6 hours. Overdoses should be treated as poisonings.

Long-term Treatment

Rarely if ever needed, but would follow that of other psychedelics.

NUTMEG/MACE

Chemical names: Myristicum and elemicin

Category: Not scheduled

Product names: Myristica fragrans, myristicum, mada shunda

Street names: None encountered

Description: Nutmeg is a hard, dark-brown nut, oval in shape and about 1 to 1-1/2 inches long. The interior is mottled dark brown and tan and of a uniform density. The nut can be grated and is usually sold in this form. Mace is a bright crimson network that covers the seed. It is usually ground into an orange-crimson powder for sale.

Means of ingestion: Both are ground or grated and mixed with liquids, often coffee, and drunk.

General Information

Both nutmeg and mace come from the nutmeg tree, *Myristica fragrans*, which grows throughout the Malayan archipelago of the East Indies. A magnificent specimen of it grows in Rick Seymour's front yard in Sausalito, California. When ripe, the fruit of this 30 to 40 foot tree resembles an apricot. Its seed is the nutmeg, while the bright crimson membrane covering the seed is processed into mace. Both have similar chemical structure and similar psychoactive properties.

In our own culture, nutmeg and mace are spices that can be found in most kitchens, usually with the cinnamon and cloves. Mace is most often used in cooking pastries, while nutmeg is sprinkled on custard or eggnog at the holiday season. One jar or tin of it may last a lifetime in the ordinary household.

Arab physicians catalogued the therapeutic uses of nutmeg as early as the seventh century, as a remedy for digestive disorders, kidney disease, pain, and lymphatic ailments. It is still considered an aphrodisiac in Yemen and consumed by men there to increase virility. In Hindu medicine, it has been prescribed for fever, consumption, asthma, and heart disease. Traditional Malayan medicine cites nutmeg for treating madness as well. In East Indian folk medicine, nutmeg is used as an analgesic painkiller and sedative. In small doses, it is used as a quieting agent for irritable children. Near the end of the 19th century, nutmeg had a brief vogue in England and America when it was mistakenly thought to bring on overdue menstruation and induce abortion (Weil, 1971).

The essential oils of nutmeg are chemically related to several of the methoxylated amphetamines. The main active ingredient of *Myristicum-* can be made into MMDA (3-methoxy-4, 5-methylenedioxyamphet- amine), while another nutmeg component, elemicin, is related to TMA (trimethoxyamphetamine) (Grinspoon & Bakalar, 1979). The structural chemical relation between nutmeg and these methoxylated amphetamines is similar to the relation between ergotamine and LSD-25.

Although both nutmeg and mace have some psychoactive qualities in their own right, the effective dosages are high, the concoctions taste terri- ble to most people, the mixtures are toxic, and the user typically sustains a painful hangover the next day. Most people who try nutmeg out of curiosity never come back for a second try (Weil & Rosen, 1983).

The psychotropic effects can range from a mild sense of floating and euphoria similar to that produced by marijuana, to major psychotomi- metic delirium. The onset of these effects can range from 10 minutes to 4 hours and their duration between 4 and 24 hours. While the intensity of the effects may be dose related, descriptions by users indicate a wide range of individual sensitivity to the effects.

General psychedelic experimentation with nutmeg and mace took place in the early 1960s, when curiosity about consciousness-changing drugs was high and LSD not yet generally available. The earliest users appar- ently found out about nutmeg's psychoactive properties from ornithologi- cal writings that described large birds, such as peacocks, as becoming drunk and staggering about after eating the nuts. Today, nutmeg abuse most commonly occurs in prisons, where other intoxicants are unavail- able. Occasional cases of nutmeg toxicity do occur, however, among young, drug naive experimenters.

Dangers

Use can cause nausea, dizziness, headaches, anxiety, or full-blown delirium. Side effects may include abdominal spasm, constipation, tach- ycardia, insomnia, and drowsiness. Overdose can produce strain on the kidneys and prolonged states of delirium. Chronic use may produce a psychotic reaction similar to stimulant psychosis.

There is one report of a fatal overdose in toxicological literature, and there are two cases of prolonged psychotic reactions. In most cases, how- ever, the hangover and kidney-pain reaction and the awful taste itself, tend to discourage subsequent experimentation.

Emergency Treatment

Acute adverse reactions, similar to those encountered with other psy- chedelic drugs, can best be countered with LSD-type talk-down techniques. These include reassurance, rest, and decrease of sensory input. In extreme cases, the patient should be treated for poisoning and sedative-hypnotic drugs used to counter the anxiety effects.

Long-term Treatment

Psychotic reactions can be treated similarly to amphetamine or stimulant psychosis. Abstinence is essential.

PHENCYCLIDINE

Chemical name: 1-(phencyclohexyl) piperidine

Category: Schedule I

Product names: Phenyclidine, ketamine, Sernylan®

Street names: PCP, peace, krystal, angel dust, hog, Captain Crunch, "THC," PeaCe, K, etc.

Description: In its basic state, phencyclidine is a white chrystalline powder with a minty, metallic taste and "chemical" smell when smoked. Phencyclidine has been sold in a variety of forms as a drug of deception for LSD, mescaline, THC, and psilocybin and, mixed with marijuana as "superweed."

Means of ingestion: The drug can be eaten, injected, and snorted. It is often mixed with dried parsley, marijuana, or tobacco and smoked.

General Information

Phencyclidine (PCP) is a dissociative anesthetic with a wide range of effects on the central nervous system. These include mind-body dissociation, anesthesia, psychomotor stimulation, and the effects generally associated with hallucinogenic drugs.

Phencyclidine was first synthesized in 1958 and tested as a human anesthetic. Side effects such as postoperative excitation, fearful delusions, and psychotic behavior made this use impractical. As Sernylan®, the drug was used by veterinarians to anesthetize large primates. A curious sidelight on this use is a recent flareup of aggressive behavior among Western grizzly bears that has been theoretically attributed to their being drugged with a form of phencyclidine during zoological studies.

Phencyclidine first emerged as a street drug in 1967 at a music festival in the Golden Gate Park panhandle in San Francisco. This occurred less than a block from the Haight-Ashbury Free Medical Clinic's psychedelic treatment center, where the first victims of the drug were taken for treatment. Called the PeaCe Pill, the drug was not well accepted at that time (Smith, 1980).

For about ten years afterward, PCP appeared primarily as an active ingredient in drugs of deception. These were usually sold to the young and nonstreetwise as LSD, mescaline, and tetrahydrocannabinol (THC) in pill and capsule form, soaked into freeze-dried mushrooms and sold as psilocybin, or mixed with marijuana and called superweed.

In the late 1970s PCP emerged as a drug of choice under such names as peace and krystal, and its horrors became an overnight media sensation. John Morgan, MD, and his associate Doreen Kagan said of it, "PCP is the ideal American-television dramatic drug because it fits so many violent stereotypes" (Morgan & Kagan, 1980).

The unpredictable behavior of PCP abusers can be frightening and dangerous. Equally frightening is the potential for overreaction by law enforcement and treatment people when confronted by PCP psychosis.

We had hoped that this drug was on the decline in the early 1980s, although its use had lingered on among the very poor at low dosage for intoxication. Recent flareups of high-dose abuse along the northeastern seaboard and the West Coast however, indicate that PCP may be with us for a long time to come.

Dangers

Our clinical findings show four different types of PCP intoxication:

1. Acute toxicity, occurring as a direct result of PCP intoxication, can involve combativeness, catatonia, convulsions, and coma. It may occur within minutes or hours of ingestion. Hypertensive crises severe enough to be fatal are rare but have been recorded. Mind-body detachment and "moon-walking" (users look as though they were trying to walk on the moon in a space suit) are common. At high doses, grand mal seizures and coma require hospitalization. Acute toxicity can last from a few minutes to 24 hours.

2. Toxic psychosis may follow repeated high-dose PCP abuse and represents a break from reality that can last from 24 hours to 7 days or more. Symptoms include impaired judgment, paranoid delusions with agitation and acting out, auditory and visual hallucinations, and behavior that is destructive to self and others.

3. Phencyclidine-precipitated psychotic episodes can follow single-dose administration of PCP and can last a month or longer. They can occur even after one use of PCP and probably involve the triggering of an underlying psychological condition. The symptoms are like those of

schizophrenia, with paranoid features and thought disorder of varying intensity.

4. Phencyclidine-induced depression may follow any of the other three stages and can last from one day to several months. Usually, this depression is a result of chronic PCP abuse. It appears to be a physically based cerebral dysfunction, manifesting a depression that can lead to suicide attempts, the abuse of other drugs in attempts to self-medicate the depression, and the resumption of PCP use (Smith, 1981).

One of the greatest concerns with PCP abuse is the violent reaction that involves irrational and destructive behavior. Bizarre violent reactions to the drug have occurred with some individuals, and although these have been overemphasized in the media, they are among the adverse effects of PCP.

Being a dissociative anesthetic, PCP renders a user's body insensible to pain during the period of intoxication. This has given rise to a street belief — especially subscribed to by enforcement officers — that people in this state have superhuman strength and maniacal powers, including the ability to break out of handcuffs and other restraints. These beliefs and a lack of clear understanding of the drug's effects contribute to a climate of fear and overreaction when dealing with PCP abusers. Also, people in this state are likely to burn or bruise themselves badly by accident, or even to break bones in their hands or feet without being aware of the pain until the drug wears off. By that time, infection may have set in, or the broken bones may have become compound fractures, causing extensive internal damage and bleeding.

There is also a delayed reaction with PCP that has been called a "flashback" but is not the same thing that is encountered with marijuana or LSD and other psychedelics. In the case of these drugs, flashback appears to be a psychological or perceptual phenomenon that can occur after the drug has completely left the system. With PCP, the recurrence of intoxication is due to the drugs being retained in the system.

Days or even weeks after the PCP trip, with no warning, the user may suddenly develop all the symptoms of acute PCP intoxication for an hour or so. This phenomenon appears to be due to the drug's extremely slow rate of elimination from the body. It travels as far as the lower intestine, but from there it is reabsorbed into the bloodstream. This reabsorption cycle causes it to recirculate periodically back through the bloodstream for days or weeks after ingestion. Also, the drug is fat soluble and will remain dormant in fat cells for a long time. Unlike the metabolites of marijuana, which enter fat cells but are no longer psychoactive, the PCP thus absorbed retains all its potency. Since PCP is highly attracted to acidic fluids, it can periodically reenter the user's spinal fluid, reenter the brain, and cause another PCP trip.

Emergency Treatment

If the user is unconscious, the first level of consideration is stabilization of the cardiovascular and respiratory systems and protection of the individual from bodily harm, such as during convulsions.

Cardiovascular system. Treatment of the hypertension with diazoxide (Hyperstat® has been recommended).

Convulsions may occur and are not necessarily limited to one or two. Recommended treatment is administration of intravenous diazepam (Valium®) over a period of two minutes following the seizure.

Occurrence of respiratory depression is unusual with pure PCP except at very high dosages. However, respiratory depression may be marked when PCP is combined with alcohol, other sedative-hypnotics, or opiates. If respiration is sufficiently depressed, mechanical respiratory assistance is necessary.

Conscious users in acute toxicity states may present with symptoms of paranoia, agitation, thought disorder, negativism, hostility, and grossly altered body image. Assaultive and antisocial behaviors are often responsible for bringing the individuals to the attention of treatment personnel. In the management of such clients, Luisada and Brown (1976) have delineated the immediate goals of treatment as follow:

- Prevention of injury to the client and others
- Assurance of continuing treatment
- Reduction of stimuli
- Amelioration of the psychosis
- Reduction of agitation

The reduction of external stimulation through the use of seclusion or a "quiet room" is of prime importance. Clinicians disagree about the most appropriate pharmacological intervention. Chlorpromazine (Thorazine®) and haloperidol have been recommended. We have preferred diazepam (Valium®) for symptomatic or behavioral control.

In any event, the user should be exposed to a minimum of external stimulation. Attempts can be made to aid excretion of the PCP. Acidification of the urine with ascorbic acid, cranberry juice, or other acidic substances can help. Phencyclidine is recycled through the enterohepatic circulation, and introducing a slurry of activated charcoal into the intestine may decrease reabsorption of PCP from the small intestine (Seymour et al., 1982).

Long-term Treatment

After the acute PCP toxicity phase has passed, some individuals develop a prolonged toxic psychosis. Most clinicians recommend the use of nonphenothiazine tranquilizers such as haloperidol. Some clinicians use sedative-hypnotic medication. There is no sound research basis for the use of either of these medications, nor is there any indication that these medications shorten the course of acute PCP toxic psychosis. It does appear, however, that they make the client more manageable in a ward, which is probably the major reason that these medications are used.

In this and other long-term treatment, probably the most effective approach is intensive counseling that includes the reassurance that the drug is still affecting the individual and that, with abstinence, all symptoms will eventually go away.

Phencyclidine-precipitated psychotic episodes are of the schizoaffective type with paranoid features and a waxing and waning thought disorder. A majority of individuals suffering these episodes have psychotic or prepsychotic personalities, and this is the major prognostic indicator. Immediate goals of treatment are the same as those listed in emergency treatment above, including prevention of injury and reduction of stimuli.

Phencyclidine-induced depression is a very common condition, the diagnosis of which is often missed, especially when it comes after PCP-precipitated psychotic reaction. In this depression, the individual has high suicide liability or may use other types of drugs to alleviate the depression. If antidepressants are prescribed on an outpatient basis, dosages for only 2 or 3 days should be dispensed at one time. The patient should be cautioned about possible interaction of tricyclic antidepressants with PCP, alcohol, and other drugs and advised to discontinue the tricyclic antidepressants if PCP use is resumed. The underlying basis of a PCP-induced depression is unknown, and disagreement exists among experienced clinicians about what constitutes the most appropriate treatment.

PSILOCIN AND PSILOCYBIN

Chemical name: 4-hydroxydimethyltryptamine — psilocybin is the phosphate ester

Category: Schedule I

Product names: None

Street names: Magic mushrooms, 'shrooms, tonanacatl, "flesh of the Gods"

Description: Indigenous to a variety of fresh and dried mushrooms. Flesh is unsually white or bluish-white. Also sold as a powder, the color is dependent on substances mixed with it. The mycellium, that part of the mushroom complex that is roughly analogous to roots in a plant, may be sold in the growing medium such as cooked rice, caked marijuana, or well-rotted wood cellulose. The mushroom spores are sold for home growing.

Means of ingestion: The mushrooms may be eaten raw, cooked into any recipe that calls for mushrooms, or steeped into a tea. The powder is eaten, insufflated, or swallowed in gelatin capsules. The mycelium is sometimes smoked along with its medium.

General Information

The chemical psilocybin is found in over 75 different species of mushrooms. These species belong to three genera: *Psilocybe*, *Panaeolus*, and *Conocybe*. These genera should not be confused with other fungi, such as *Amanita muscaria* and *Amanita pantherina*, which derive their psychoactive effects from muscimole, an alkaloid that may be physically dangerous at high doses (Grinspoon & Bakalar, 1979).

Appearing in a wide variety of shapes, sizes, and potencies, psilocybin-containing mushrooms can be found in most parts of the world. Fifteen species have been identified in the Pacific Northwest of America alone (Weil, 1981).

Although the ritualistic use of these mushrooms has been traced back as far as 1000 B.C. in Pre-Columbian Mexico (Wasson, 1972), and their use continued in secret after its suppression by the Spanish Inquisition, these mushrooms and their effects were considered a myth by Western medicine until they were "rediscovered" in the mid-1950s. At that time they were still being used clandestinely by shamans of the Oaxacan Indians.

This rediscovery of psilocybin preceded the epidemic of psychedelic drug use in the Western world by a few years. In the early 1960s, experimenters made pilgrimages to the highlands of Mexico to participate in "magic mushroom" ceremonies. Mycology, the study of mushrooms, became popular, and young mycologists discovered that these psychedelic mushrooms could be found just about anywhere. Illustrated guides and handbooks (Stamets, 1978; Menser, 1977) have had wide distribution, and growing kits with mushroom spores and instructions are available in many states.

A derivative of tryptamine, psilocybin is converted, when ingested, to psilocin, which is also present in the mushrooms. Both substances are classified as "indole" hallucinogens and are similar to LSD and serotonin, an internal neurotransmitter (chemical messenger) that affects many central nervous system functions (Chilton et al., 1979). These drugs probably work by stimulating serotonin receptor sites in the brain.

The effects of psilocybin are roughly similar to those of LSD, peyote, and mescaline but are often considered more gentle than these. Although dosage varies among mushroom types, general potency is about 200 times less than that of LSD. Tolerance develops rapidly, and there is cross-tolerance with LSD and mescaline. Effects are usually apparent within a half hour and may last from 4 to 8 hours.

Setting and attitude of the consumer have a great influence on effect. Most psilocybin users report complex cognitive changes in sight, hearing, taste and touch — all regarded as altered states of consciousness. Colors may seem brighter; closed-eye visual patterns are likely. Sounds can appear richer, and a crossing of senses — i.e., seeing sounds and hearing colors — may occur (Grinspoon & Bakalar, 1979).

With the exception of very high doses, the user is usually aware that these are drug effects and is not threatened by them. Users may feel an overwhelming sense of lightness and a sense that all is essentially right with themselves and the universe. Unlike LSD, psilocybin is not associated with a postexperience energy letdown.

Dangers

Psilocybin can cause anxiety, depression, disorientation, and dissociation with reality, especially at excessive dosages, as a result of fear of the drug's effects, or in response to inappropriate settings such as rock concerts. Prolonged psychotic reactions are rare and usually occur where psychological problems already exist (Beck & Dale, 1982). Toxicity occurs at about 2000 times the normally effective dose. Problems have developed from adolescents using psilocybin as part of a polydrug abuse pattern. Mixing with alcohol is not a good idea, nor is driving or operating machinery while intoxicated.

Emergency Treatment

A talk-down similar to that used for bad LSD trips is effetive for severe reactions. Talk-downs should be supportive, nonjudgmental, and comforting. In extreme cases, low doses of minor tranquilizers such as Librium® or Valium® may be used. External stimulation should be limited, and the individual should lie down and relax.

Poisonous Varieties

Some mushroom species thought to be poisonous do resemble some psilocybin mushrooms. Someone who has eaten the "wrong mushroom" should be taken to an emergency room or poison center with a sample of the mushroom if possible. The staff should be aware that large doses of atropine (an outmoded treatment for mushroom poisoning) can potentiate the effects of muscimole and do damage rather than help.

MISCELLANEOUS PSYCHEDELICS/ PSYCHOTOMIMETICS/HALLUCINOGENICS

Many drugs in all the categories have some psychedelic, psychotomimetic, and/or hallucinogenic qualities, and a number of substances throughout the world have some consciousness effectiveness. Several miscellaneous substances that are usually counted among these drugs are listed below.

Harmala Alkaloids

The harmala alkaloids include harmine, harmaline, and *d*-1,2,3,4-tetrahydroharmine. They are found in the Near Eastern shrub *Peganum harmala* or Syrian rue, the bark of South American *Banisteriopsis* vines, and the vine *Tetrapterys methystica*. The bark of these South American vines is made into a drink known variously as ayahuasca (vine of the souls), caapi, natema, pinde, yage, and kahi. Taken in liquid form or as snuff, these drugs have a duration of 4 to 8 hours. Physical effects include nausea, vomiting, sweating, dizziness, tremors, and numbness. Users report trancelike states with vivid images involving color enhancement, usually in the blue-green range, and a wide range of emotional response. Cultural images seem to dominate, but there is some discussion as to whether the drug has influenced the culture or vice versa.

Ibogaine

Ibogaine is an alkaloid found in the root of the West African plant *Tabernanthe iboga*, used primarily as a stimulant and aphrodisiac when taken at low dosages, but resembling the harmala alkaloids when used ceremonially at high dosages. Physical and psychological effects are similar to those of harmaline. Effective at psychedelic doses for 8 to 12 hours.

N, N-Dimethyltryptamine (DMT)

DMT is structurally similar to psilocybin and is present in hallucinogenic drinks of South American shrubs, including *Mimosa hostilis*. In the United States, it has been smoked after being soaked into parsley or other smokable substances, taken in liquid form, or injected either intravenously or intramuscularly. The effects are similar to those of LSD, but sympathomimetic effects such as dilated pupils, raised blood pressure, and elevated pulse rate are more pronounced. The most unique quality of this drug is its rapidity of effect. Effects can be experienced within seconds of injection, peak in 5 to 20 minutes, and often end within half an hour.

Muscimole

One of a family of alkaloids known collectively as isoxazoles, this drug is found in *Amanita muscaria*, the fly agaric mushroom. This fungus has a bright-red to orange cap dotted with what looks like spots of cottage cheese. Muscimole is also found in the rarer *Amanita pantherina*. These mushrooms grow in high temperate regions throughout the world. Effects include muscle spasms, trembling, nausea, loss of equilibrium, dizziness, and numbness. Subjective patterns include a trancelike half-sleep with visions followed by elation, feelings of lightness and physical strength, heightened sense perception, synesthesia, and body-image changes. At high doses, the drug can cause delirium, coma, and amnesia, making this a potentially dangerous drug. The effects last about 6 hours. The *Amanita muscaria* gained some notoriety in the late 1960s when several mycologists/historians postulated that its ritual use may have been responsible for much of early Christian mysticism.

Anticholinergic Hallucinogens

A group of drugs that are included within the psychedelic listing, the anticholinergic hallucinogens are often regarded as classic poisons as well as hallucinogens. Historically, they have had a variety of medical as well as political indications ranging from use as cold remedy ingredients to agents for assassination.

Atropa Belladonna

Atropine was isolated from *Atropa belladonna* (deadly nightshade) in 1831. In keeping with its morbid origin, the name atropine was derived from Atropos, the Greek fate who cut everyone's thread of life. It was used by medieval witches to induce a feeling of flying. It also had a reputation as an aphrodisiac.

Mandragora Officinarum

The mandrake plant also contains an atropine-like substance, and its psychoactive qualities are noted in the Bible. In ancient times, it was used medically to treat pain and stress.

Hyoscyamus Niger

Also known as henbane, *Hyosyamus niger* contains scopolamine and *l*-lysocyamine. Less popular than mandrake, it was also used in the Middle Ages. It is thought to be the drug that poisoned Hamlet's father.

Datura

Datura is a worldwide species of plants that contains atropine, scopolamine, and hyoscyamine in varying amounts. Its medicinal use was recorded in China far back into ancient times.

Collectively, these drugs have been used for thousands of years in shamanistic and magical practices as well as for medical problems. Their potency and dangers are so pronounced that they tend not to represent a drug abuse problem.

In their book *Psychedelic Drugs Reconsidered* (1979), Lester Grinspoon, MD, and James B. Bakalar point out that similar consciousness changes are not only caused by a wide variety of drugs but by a widely divergent variety of nondrug experience as well. In this section, we have discussed the substances that are usually considered psychedelic, psychotomimetic, and/or hallucinogenic, but it should be noted, as these authors aver, that "the same drug can produce many different reactions, and the same reaction can be produced by many different drugs." At varying times and in varying circumstances nearly every substance discussed in this book has produced some sort of mystical experience. Further, similar experiences have been encountered in such states as "dreams, psychosis, starvation, isolation, high fever, . . . hypnotic trance, repetitive chanting, prolonged wakefulness, revivalist exhortation, song or dance, fasting, hyperventilation, special postures, exercises and techniques for concentrating attention."

Narcotic Antagonists

NALOXONE HYDROCHLORIDE
AND NALTREXONE HYDROCHLORIDE

Chemical names: N-allyl-noroxymorphone and N-cyclopropylmethyl-noroxymorphone

Category: Not psychoactive substances, not scheduled

Product names: Narcan® and Trexan® respectively

Street names: None noted

Description: Naloxone is available in liquid form in 1 ml ampules, 10 ml multiple dose vials, and 1 ml prefilled disposable syringes.
Naltrexone comes in 50 mg round tablets, scored and imprinted with DuPont on one side and TREXAN® on the other.

Means of ingestion: Naloxone is injected. Naltrexone is swallowed.

General Information

Naloxone and naltrexone are narcotic antagonists. They have no psychoactive effects. What they do is block the opiate receptor sites in the brain and by doing so block all the effects of the narcotics that use these receptor sites. These substances are ineffective in blocking such other drugs as sedative-hypnotics, stimulants, or psychedelics.
In recent years it has been learned that opiate narcotics such as Darvon®, codeine, morphine, and heroin, as well as a number of synthethic opioid analgesics, form their connection to the central nervous system by occupying opiate receptor sites at neural synapses. The normal function of these sites is to facilitate the action of such internal agents as endorphins, which are produced by such activities as physical exercise or pain and have positive effects similar to those of opiates. Endorphins or external opiates work in these sites in a way similar to a key fitting into a lock or a plug in a socket. It is this occupation of and manipulation of the

receptor sites that gives rise to the effects we recognize as narcotic: euphoria, drowsiness, a sense of well-being, and pain reduction. Stimulation of these sites results in opiate intoxication, and if sufficiently increased, opiate overdose. There are multiple sites on these receptors,
with external opiates such as heroin occupying some and internal opiates
such as endorphins occupying others.

Two recent events have brought narcotic antagonists into public attention. In 1983, the manufacturers of Talwin®, a synthetic painkiller, added
naloxone to its preparation. They did this to discourage the injecting of a
Talwin/tripelennamine combination as a substitute for heroin. Although
naloxone and naltrexone have similar effects, there are some marked differences between the two.

Naloxone

Naloxone has long been part of the emergency drug treatment pharmacopeia. When it is used to reverse the effects of a narcotic, the results can
be truly miraculous and life saving. Anyone who has seen a semicomatose and fading victim of narcotic overdose come back to consciousness — full consciousness within moments of a Narcan® injection — has
seen a medical miracle.

Narcan® acts by removing opiate molecules from their binding sites —
it literally "kicks them out" of the receptors and takes their place. This
substitution reverses the effects and keeps the opiate molecules in the
open bloodstream (where they can have no effect on the central nervous
system) until they can be metabolized and excreted without causing further harm.

This antagonist is short-acting and short lived. Therefore, if the overdose victim has taken a long-acting narcotic such as methadone, the Nar-
can® must be readministered when symptoms of intoxication begin to
reappear. Otherwise, the long-acting opiate would reoccupy the receptors
and the victim would go back into overdose.

Because naloxone must be injected to be effective — it is destroyed by
stomach acids — it was considered ideal for adding to Talwin®. Talwin®
is the trade name for pentazocine, the painkiller with a potency roughly
similar to that of codeine. It comes in pill form and is supposed to be
swallowed. When Talwin® is crushed with tripelennamine, an antihistamine with both stimulant and depressant effects, and injected, the result
is said to simulate a heroin-cocaine "speedball." This mixture was called
"T's and Blues." In the new preparation, however, the naloxone blocks
the effects of the Talwin® if it is injected, but not if it is swallowed.

Naltrexone

By contrast, naltrexone is effective when swallowed. It is also much longer acting than naloxone. A dose of 50 mg of naltrexone effectively blocks the primary effects of any opiate dose for 24 hours. A 150 mg dose provides blockage for up to 72 hours. If a narcotic is used while the naltrexone dose is in effect, there is no euphoria, no respiratory depression, no relief of pain — no response whatsoever (Ling & Wesson, 1980).

On the surface, then, naltrexone would seem an ideal means of warding off recidivism — relapse among clean opiate abusers. Unlike the alcoholic who uses Antabuse®, opiate users do not get violently ill if they try to use the drug. With naltrexone, there is no adverse reaction: There is no reaction at all. Drug cravings and drug-seeking behavior are reduced when the user knows that the drug will have no effect.

One drawback is immediately obvious. That is the difficulty of getting any but the most dedicated, recovery-motivated patient to agree to this treatment in the first place. Naltrexone should be viewed as an adjunct to recovery while the patient is encouraged to participate in a recovery group to learn to live a comfortable and responsible life without the use of drugs.

Research has indicated that naltrexone can be an effective aid to recovery in narcotic addiction when used with certain willing and highly motivated patients (Ginzburg, 1984). Treatment researcher Donald R. Wesson, MD (1984), characterizes patients as opiate abusers if they:

- Do not meet criteria for methadone maintenance
- Cannot take methadone because of job considerations
- Have done well on and want to withdraw from methadone
- Select naltrexone as an alternative to methadone

Programs involved in this therapy would be well monitored, outpatient programs issuing the antagonist in 72-hour-dosage pills as an adjunct to other treatment.

Dangers

There are three basic difficulties in the clinical use of naltrexone (Wesson, 1984):

1. Acute narcotic withdrawal will occur if naltrexone is taken by an opiate-dependent person who has not been fully detoxified prior to its use. Symptoms may include drug craving, anxiety, drug-seeking behavior, yawning, perspiration, lacrimation, rhinorrhea, broken sleep, mydriasis, gooseflesh, muscle twitches, hot flashes and chills, bone and muscle aches, anorexia, insomnia, low grade fever, motor restlessness,

weakness, abdominal cramps, nausea, vomiting, diarrhea, weight loss, and increases in respiration, pulse, and blood pressure. In other words, all the symptoms of narcotic withdrawal.

2. Acute pain management in injured naltrexone-maintained patients will require ingenuity by the treating physician, as the antagonist will block narcotic analogues.

3. Maintenance patients having elective surgery need to stop their dose 72 hours before surgery and not start again until 72 hours after their last dose of narcotic. To avoid relapse, naltrexone should be restarted before the patient leaves the hospital.

The greatest danger with naloxone is that of allowing a patient who has overdosed on a long-acting narcotic to lapse back into overdose.

Emergency Treatment

Acute withdrawal precipitated by naltrexone being used by a not fully detoxified opiate addict is not life threatening but should be closely monitored, with therapy tailored to meet individual needs. Significant fluid losses from vomiting and diarrhea may require intravenous fluid administration (Klebern, 1984).

In injuries to patients on naltrexone maintenance, pain from arms and legs can be managed with nerve blocks. Trauma or surgery to the head or torso is more difficult. Ketamine can be effective. In an emergency situation requiring analgesia in which relief can be achieved only with opioids, the amount of opioid required may be greater than usual, and the resulting respiratory depression may be deeper and more prolonged. In such circumstances, a rapidly acting analgesic that minimizes respiratory depression is preferred. The amount of analgesic administered should be titrated to the needs of the patient. Whatever drug is used, the patient should be monitored closely by appropriately trained personnel in a hospital setting. It should also be noted that use of an opioid analgesic may promote nonreceptor-mediated actions that can result in facial swelling, itching, and other histamine reactions.

Psychoactive Drug Combinations

GLUTETHIMIDE AND CODEINE

Chemical names: Glutethimide is 2-ethyl-2-phenylglutarimide. Codeine is methylmorphine.

Category: Codeine is Schedule II. Glutethimide is Schedule II.

Product names: Glutethimide (Doriden®). Codeine occurs in many analgesic combinations but is usually mentioned therein by name, for example, Codeine & Empirin, Phenergan VC Expectorant w/Codeine, etc.

Street names: Set-ups, loads, doors, four-doors

Description: Both drugs come in tablet form.

Means of ingestion: Intravenous injection.

General Information

Glutethimide (Doriden®) is a nonbarbiturate sedative-hypnotic used in treating nonchronic insomnia. Codeine is an opium derivative used as a general painkiller. Both drugs are Schedule II – i.e., used medically but bearing a high abuse potential and calling for controlled, triplicate prescription. They are not meant to be combined.

The combination of glutethimide and codeine is supposed to simulate the effects of heroin and is available only on the illicit street market. Owing to the danger involved in use at an intoxicating quantity, we feel that there is no recreational use of this combination – only abuse. First seen in early 1980, the abuse of set-ups escalated toward the end of 1980. At the Haight-Ashbury Free Medical Clinic we saw an increase in both drug overdose and drug dependence associated with set-ups. In southern California, the same combination is called "loads" (Marder, 1981).

Dangers

This is a particularly dangerous combination for overdose because it combines a narcotic with a potent sedative-hypnotic that approximates in lethality a short-acting barbiturate. Glutethimide can be deadly at only 5 to 10 times the therapeutic dose used to induce sleep. In some persons, glutethimide produces an atypical intoxication seizure. Daily use in excess of 30 days at a level 5 times the therapeutic level can produce physical dependence. Chronic use may cause stumbling, staggering, and neurological deficits in hands and legs that can progress to paralysis. Psychiatric problems may be precipitated or aggravated.

High doses of the aspirin and acetaminophen found in codeine compounds can cause gastric ulcers, tinnitus, and hearing loss, as well as liver damage and blood coagulation disorders. Other additives in high quantity can cause kidney damage, central nervous system (CNS) problems, and death.

Emergency Treatment

Owing to the nature of glutethimide as a short-acting sedative-hypnotic, there is no specific antagonist for either overdose or dependence. Both conditions require the expertise and facilities of an emergency room, hospital dependency unit, drug treatment clinic, or poison control center. Treatment personnel need to know that these drugs are involved so that all proper life-sustaining measures can be taken.

The overdose is only partially reversed by the administration of naloxone (Narcan®), which, as a narcotic antagonist, will nullify only the effects of the codeine. The effects of the glutethimide must be managed conservatively until it is excreted from the body. A life-support system for both respiration and the cardiovascular system is often necessary. Vigorous medical intervention is indicated, and hospitalization is usually required.

Long-term Treatment

Withdrawal from codeine dependence by itself is similar to all other opiate withdrawal. That is, it is not life threatening and can be carried out in a variety of outpatient modalities. Glutethimide withdrawal is much more complex than detoxification from codeine. It can induce seizures, withdrawal psychosis, or death. The withdrawal syndrome is similar to that seen after the abrupt cessation of a short-acting barbiturate. At the Haight-Ashbury Free Medical Clinic and allied inpatient facilities, we have used a phenobarbital substitution and withdrawal technique for glutethimide dependence with good results. A sedative dose of phenobarbital (30 mg) is substituted for each 250 mg of glutethimide. After two days' stabilization on the phenobarbital, the phenobarbital dosage is reduced 30 mg a day. Variations include (1) the substitution of another short-acting barbiturate followed by graded reduction of dosage or (2) graded reduction of the glutethimide itself. We believe, however, that these techniques are less effective, and the dosages are harder to titrate. Any of these techniques should only be used on an inpatient basis.

During the withdrawal phase, attention should be given to the possibility of phenobarbital intoxication and to possible manipulative behavior by the patient in a effort to get more medication. The latter, if successful, can greatly impede the progress of detoxification and does not help the patient. If signs of intoxication are observed, the dosage of the substitution drug is reduced. Because of the potential for seizure, glutethimide withdrawal or any sedative-hypnotic withdrawal should never be treated without medication in a "cold turkey" fashion, nor should it be attempted by inexperienced personnel.

TALWIN® AND TRIPELENNAMINE (PYRIBENZAMINE)

Chemical names: Talwin® is a combination of pentazocine hydrochloride (Pc) and naloxone hydrochloride (Nh). Pc is 1,2,3,4,5,6-hexahydro-6, 11-dimethyl-3-(3-methyl-2-butenyl)-2, 6-methano-3-benzazocin-8-ol hydrochloride. Nh is Morpinan-6-one,4,5,epoxy-3,14-dihydroxy-17(2-propenyl)-,hydrochloride,(5a) — . Tripelennamine is 2-(benzyl *l*2-(dimethylamino)ethyl-*l*-amino) pyridine.

Category: Talwin® is Schedule IV, tripelennamine unscheduled.

Product names: Talwin®, Talwin NX®, PBZ, PBZ-SR, Pyribenzamine

Street names: T's and Blues, T's and B's, Tops and Bottoms, Toms and Bettys, Tricycles and Bicycles, etc.

Description: Tripelennamine hydrochloride is an antihistamine occurring as a white, crystalline powder that slowly darkens on exposure to light and is freely soluble in water and alcohol. Talwin® is an analgesic that appears as a white crystalline substance soluble in acidic aqueous solutions.

Means of ingestion: Both drugs come in pill form but are crushed, dissolved in water and injected intravenously.

General Information

Talwin® is the trade name for pentazocine, a synthetic analgesic with a potency roughly equivalent to codeine. Tripelennamine is an antihistamine with both stimulant and depressant effects. The combination of these drugs was used experimentally for the symptomatic relief of narcotic withdrawal symptoms. In medical use they are taken orally. Both drugs have a history of individual abuse, but abuse by injection in combination appeared first in the Chicago area in the early 1970s.

The effects of T's and Blues are reported to be similar to those of a heroin-cocaine "speedball." Users report a "rush" similar to that experienced on injecting heroin and a consistency of effect—as opposed to street heroin, which may fluctuate greatly depending on purity.

The Talwin®/tripelennamine may turn out to be an example of drug abuse control by the pharmaceutical industry. In an effort to fight abuse through injection, the manufacturers of Talwin® have added naloxone to the formula. Naloxone (Narcan®) is a narcotic antagonist used to reverse heroin overdoses. It is destroyed by stomach acid so that when Talwin® with naloxone is taken orally it still has the desired analgesic effect. However, if the drug is injected, the antagonist occupies the receptor sites and prevents any narcotic effect from taking place. There are some dangers; for example, abusers may raise the dosage in order to override the antagonist and end up with a sedative-hypnotic overdose, or they may go into narcotic withdrawal. Nevertheless, this move by the manufacturer may eliminate one of the more pernicious drug abuse combinations. Similar combinations may appear in the future, however.

Dangers

The drug combination, and Talwin® itself, are physically addicting and will produce some withdrawal symptoms. These appear to be milder than heroin withdrawal symptoms and easier to treat. Users of this combination become compulsive in their drug-taking and drug-seeking behavior in the same way as heroin abusers.

The greatest danger may be from inert ingredients. Irritants in the chemicals, and buffers that stay in solution despite users' attempts to filter them out, can cause extensive soft-tissue destruction. Abscesses, scars, and "woody edema"—hard knotty areas in veins that infect easily—are common. Deep-muscle and tendon damage is also common. Severe tightening of major joints (hip and shoulder) can result in an inability to move, and in some cases infection submerged in the tissue can require major surgery and joint replacement. Septic states and bacterial endocarditis can occur. Talc often builds up in the eye, brain, and lungs of the abuser. Accumulation in the lungs of a microcrystalline filler used in manufacturing both drugs can lead to pulmonary fibrosis, impairment of lung function, and death.

These same fillers accumulate in the eye, brain, and kidneys. Some physicians have observed a variety of neurological syndromes, including brain infections, which may result from altered brain function due to these deposits. These dire results tend to make extended use of this combination somewhat self-limiting.

Tripelennamine is cross-tolerant with alcohol and other sedative-hypnotics. Use with alcohol can institute the sedative-hypnotic additive effect and could result in a fatal overdose.

Emergency Treatment

Overdoses are rare. The Talwin® effects can be reversed with naloxone as with any other narcotic overdose. Tripelennamine overdose treatment would follow that outlined in the chapter on central nervous system depressants.

Long-term Treatment

Detoxification can use any of the methods employed in heroin detoxification. In general, detoxification is easier and shorter than with heroin. The greatest dangers with this drug combination are the cumulative deposits. In time the damage from these may be irreversible. Education about the eventual course of the problem may be the best approach.

UPPERS AND DOWNERS

One of the classic drug abuse combinations is that of a narcotic analgesic or a sedative-hypnotic with a stimulant. Many abusers discover that rather than fully canceling each other out, each tends to mediate the long-term dysphoric or undesirable effects of the other. In the short term, such combinations tend to make larger doses of each easier to handle. Upper/downer combinations fall into two abuse patterns: "speedballing" and the upper/downer series.

"Speedball"

The street name for a combination of both drugs is a "speedball." The term can be used for any combination of upper and downer taken together but is usually used for the injected combination of cocaine and heroin. The speedball was mentioned in novels of the early 20th century, including the mystery stories of Dashiel Hammett, and until recently cocaine was provided along with heroin to British maintenance patients.

The direct combining of these drugs can dangerously mask their effects. For example, the alcohol abuser may have enough alcohol to be safely passed out, but with the addition of amphetamine may be wide awake in a dangerously intoxicated condition and think himself capable of driving. Similarly, the folk remedy of trying to sober someone up with the stimulant coffee only creates a wide-awake drunk.

The speedball and its dangers received much recent publicity with the death of actor-comedian John Belushi. His death was attributed to a speedball-type overdose in which the cocaine masked the accumulating effects of heroin until too late.

Upper/Downer Series

In the second pattern, one drug type is used to mediate the long-term effects of the other. With cocaine or amphetamine use, for example, a stimulant run will in time result in feeling "wired," depressed, or even psychotic. A sedative-hypnotic, antidepressant-type drug or a narcotic will help the abuser through this jagged period. Alcohol is often used in this pattern. The most current manifestation of this pattern is the smoking of high potency heroin between runs by cocaine freebasers.

Look-alike Drugs
and Drugs of Deception

Street drugs are not always what they seem. The history of the illicit drug trade is chock-a-block with horror stories detailing the consequences to victims of misrepresented products. In the street drug market, there is no such thing as a "Food and Drug Administration" or a "Better Business Bureau." It is strictly a case of *caveat emptor* — let the buyer beware.

Misrepresented drugs fall into two general categories:

- *Look-alike drugs:* Nonscheduled substances that may resemble in appearance or effect scheduled drugs that are popular on the illicit market but hard to come by. Look-alikes may be represented as being the illegal drug or may be advertised as a legal counterpart.
- *Drugs of deception:* One scheduled drug is disguised and sold as another scheduled drug that may be hard or impossible to get, or a stronger drug is added to a weaker one to give it more potency.

LOOK-ALIKE DRUGS

The most common look-alike drugs in our society are look-alike stimulants. Amphetamine look-alikes are often manufactured to resemble the more notorious amphetamine preparations that were massively diverted into the illegal market before production cutbacks were imposed in the 1970s. Many of these look-alikes are even given the street names of their scheduled counterparts, such as "black beauties" or "pink footballs." Although these pills may initially be sold as "legal pep pills" or diet aids, they are often resold as the amphetamines that they resemble.

Contents of these pills and capsules are all legal. They include phenylpropanolamine, a nasal decongestant and appetite suppressant; ephedrine, a decongestant; and caffeine, a common stimulant found in coffee, tea, and cold pills. In the spring of 1982, it was estimated that over 90% of street amphetamines actually contained little or no amphetamine but were made up of the same ingredients as look-alikes. This included both white, round tablets with a cross cut and powdered "crank" or "speed."

Since then, the production of "cocaine substitutes" and phony cocaine has proliferated. Contents of cocaine look-alikes are usually similar to those of amphetamine look-alikes, but they often include such substances as lydocaine to mimic the numbing topical anesthetic effects of cocaine, and mannitol, an inert substance often used to cut real cocaine because it has cocaine's crystalline appearance.

Reactions to these drugs can include nervousness, insomnia, drowsiness, sharp rises in blood pressure and body heat, cerebral hermorrhages, and temporary hypertensive episodes. Anyone who is used to abusing real amphetamines would be inclined to use high dosages of look-alikes in attempting to achieve an amphetamine or cocaine "rush" and would become victim to these adverse effects that do not usually occur at normal dosages. Conversely, real amphetamines or cocaine might be mistaken for their doubles and taken to overdose amounts. Even veteran cocaine and amphetamine users can be confused and unable to tell the difference between their drug and a look-alike.

There is a further danger, especially with street speed and phony cocaine, of dangerous additives and impurities. They represent much more than consumer fraud and can, in fact, be deadly. There are no rules in street drugs. The most blatant case of this we recall was the sale at a rock concert of ground glass as cocaine. But many corrosive and highly toxic substances including Drano®, borax, and epoxy have been used in street preparations.

DRUGS OF DECEPTION

Those of us who are old enough remember stories from Prohibition of people being killed or blinded when unscrupulous bootleggers substituted wood alcohol for grain alcohol in their products. These were early instances of drugs of deception.

In the heyday of psychedelic drugs, from the mid-1960s to the mid-1970s, misrepresentation of drugs was so common that many drug users adopted a stoical attitude of "whatever gets you off so long as it doesn't kill you." Dried commercial mushrooms were dosed with LSD and sold as psilocybin. Phencyclidine (PCP) masqueraded as LSD, mescaline, and any other psychedelic that was popular at the time. Only God and the manufacturers knew what was in the pills sold as tetrahydro cannabinol. The situation was so bad that street drug analysis programs, many of them sponsored by medical testing companies, sprang up across the country. The best known of these, sponsored by PharmChem Laboratories of Palo Alto, California, continued its street-drug testing service until 1984.

Drugs of deception often take advantage of a popular drug's reputation, especially if that drug suddenly becomes hard to get. A current example is the rash of counterfeit "quaaludes" that have hit the street since the Lemmon Company ceased manufacture in 1984. The two primary components in these "ludes" are diazepam (Valium®) in high doses and phenobarbital, a long-acting barbiturate. Other ingredients have been the antihistamines peniramine and doxylamine, the pain relievers aspirin and acetaminophen, and a wide variety of other additives including other barbiturates, arthritis medicines, O-toluidine (a toxic methaqualone precursor also used in manufacturing dyes) and epoxy glue.

Obviously, there are a number of problems from these and other drugs of deception, not the least among them being the confusion caused in attempting to treat overdoses and other adverse effects. Bogus ingredients can greatly affect the treatment of withdrawal symptoms. For example, with methaqualone withdrawal, the peak liability for seizures may be the second day. With high-dose diazepam (Valium®), it is the fifth to the seventh day, and if alcohol is involved, this peak can be delayed to the ninth or tenth day after cessation of use.

These look-alike methaqualones are appearing both in the form of Quaalude® Lemmon 714s and as British Mandrax®. With the latter, they are often represented as having been smuggled in from Europe or India. Mandrax®, as manufactured overseas, is a mixture of 250 mg of methaqualone and 25 mg of diphehydramine hydrochloride, a potent antihistamine.

Some of the drugs of deception can be especially sinister. For example, there is MPPP, the phoney meperidine preparation that can cause parkinsonism through an impurity in its manufacture, and the tremendous risk of overdoses from the highly potent analogues of fentanyl that have been marketed as "china white" and other high-strength heroins. With the increasing profit motive in illicit drugs coupled with a proliferation of underground chemists whose skills range from the highly sophisticated through the sociopathic to the imbecilic, the situation will probably get worse.

EMERGENCY TREATMENT

The ongoing proliferation of both look-alikes and drugs of deception underlines the importance of correctly identifying the specific substances that have been taken by the victim. This can be done by analysis of the drug itself if a sample is still available, or by analysis of blood, urine, or stomach contents. If an opiate overdose is probable, a trial injection of naloxone (Narcan®) is indicated.

The following applies to the more common stimulant look-alikes discussed earlier:

At low doses the stimulant effects of phenylpropanolamine (PPA), ephedrine, and caffeine, the primary ingredients of legally manufactured over-the-counter diet aids, look-alikes, and street stimulant counterfeits, are relatively mild. The therapeutic ratio of these stimulant compounds, however, is narrow in that the dosage required to produce euphoria is very close to a toxic dose. If one takes several of these look-alikes to achieve a stimulant euphoria, one can also have stimulant toxicity, commonly producing acute anxiety—being "overamped." These compounds produce a good deal of physical peripheral stimulation and will produce increased pulse rate, cardiac arrhythmia, or rapid and uneven heartbeat; elevated body temperature; and elevation in blood pressure. With a massive overdose, these cardiac stimulant effects are potentially fatal. These require medical management, including the use of beta adrenergic blocking agents such as propanolol (Inderol®), which blocks these acute stimulant effects, plus other medical life support measures.

When individuals die from massive overdoses, either by accident or in a suicide, it is usually the result of cardiac arrest, hyperpyrexia (greatly elevated body temperature), and convulsions. A massive stimulant overdose represents a medical emergency and requires immediate medical attention.

If an individual uses high dosages over a long time, a stimulant psychosis may develop, as is true with any stimulant. The most extreme manifestations are characterized by paranoia with ideas of reference and auditory and visual hallucinations similar to those seen in high-dose, prolonged amphetamine or cocaine abuse. These symptoms require antipsychotic medication such as haloperidol (Haldol®), drug counseling, and often short-term psychiatric hospitalization. Lower-dose dependence usually does not require medication, but rather drug counseling.

Simple anxiety reactions with no physical symptoms can usually be managed with reassurance and the use of a sedative compound administered by mouth, such as diazepam (Valium®).

SECTION TWO:
ASPECTS OF ABUSE AND TREATMENT

Drug Abuse and Addiction: Why?

If the consequences of drug and alcohol abuse are so bad and so obvious, why do people do it? More may have been learned about addiction in the last decade than in all previous medical history, but we still have a long way to go before we can answer that simple question — Why?

What has been done in the field of substance abuse is to establish a series of paradigms, or models, of what we think may be true. These are often in conflict with one another. Abuse of and addiction to drugs is a highly emotional issue.

In the news we read that "the motorist whose 1980 killing of a 13-year-old girl set off the nationwide Mothers Against Drunk Drivers movement has been arrested again after another accident involving alcohol." MADD's founder, the mother of the girl killed five years ago, "reacted angrily." "What is the man doing drinking again?" she said. "When is he going to learn you can't drink and drive? He should be put away for life" (*Sacramento Wire*, 1985).

Can this man learn that you can't drink and drive? Should he be put away for life? Is he a moral monster, or is he the helpless victim of a potentially fatal disease?

We know philosophically that reality is affected by the observer and that how we see things has a lot to do with what we see. Definitions have had a lot to do with not only our attitudes toward substance abuse but also the way we treat substance abusers and the ways in which we regulate the availability of psychoactive drugs. Two decades ago, for example, narcotic users — popularly called "junkies" — were all considered criminals. Treatment for opiate addiction consisted of more-or-less "cold turkey" withdrawal during incarceration in federal facilities like the one in Lexington, Kentucky. When their terms were up, these "criminals" were released back into society, usually back into the subculture where their need for the drug was quickly satisfied and opiate dependence reestablished.

During this same period, therapists were finding it useful to regard alcoholism as a progressive disease, which, if left untreated, could lead to increasing biological, psychological, or social dysfunction and probable death.

In the 1960s when middle-class youth became in part a drug-using subculture, national attention was drawn to the possibility that drug abuse might be a medical as well as a moral dilemma. The federal government established a Special Action Office for Drug Abuse Prevention and then a National Institute on Drug Abuse modeled after the National Institute on Mental Health. Drug abusers were still criminals, but maybe they were "sick" criminals.

The use of drugs has now proliferated and extended across all social strata. We no longer have a drug-using subculture, we are a culture that uses drugs.

In a way we always did. There is an apocryphal account that early in his tenure, NIDA director Jerome H. Jaffe was asked at a conference of drug abuse experts to define drug abuse. He is said to have replied that drug abuse is the use, usually by self-administration, of any psychoactive drug that is not medically prescribed or indicated. It was a magic moment at conferences, 10:30 or thereabouts, and the tinkle of silver and china came from the back of the room as attendees began drifting toward the coffee urns. An attending doctor pointed out that by Dr. Jaffe's definition, most of the people in the room were about to become drug abusers. The phrase ". . . or within the social norms of a given culture" was hastily added to the definition.

But social norms change with time and vary geographically. Labeling all nonmedical drug use as abuse obscures the distinctions between compulsive abuse and occasional low-dose recreational use or experimental use of a drug because of curiosity or for circumstantial performance facilitation. The National Commission on Marihuana and Drug Abuse (1973) presented the following classifications of nonmedical drug use, taking into account that all nonmedical use may not be de facto abuse.

> *Experimental use:* A short-term nonpatterned trial of one or more drugs, motivated primarily by curiosity or a desire to experience an altered mood state.
> *Recreational use:* Occurs in a social setting among friends or acquaintances who desire to share an experience which they define as both acceptable and pleasurable. Generally, recreational use is both

voluntary and patterned and tends not to escalate to more frequent or intense use patterns.

Circumstantial use: Generally motivated by the user's perceived need or desire to achieve a new and anticipated effect in order to cope with a specific problem, situation or condition of a personal or vocational nature. This classification would include students who utilize stimulants during preparation for exams, long-distance truckers who rely on similar substances to provide extended endurance and alertness, military personnel who use drugs to cope with stress in combat situations, athletes who attempt to improve their performance, and housewives who seek to relieve tension, anxiety, boredom or other stresses through the use of sedatives or stimulants.

Intensified use: Drug use which occurs at least daily and is motivated by an individual's perceived need to achieve relief from a persistent problem or stressful situation, or his desire to maintain a certain self-prescribed level of performance. . . . A very different group of intensified users are those who have turned to drugs as sources of excitement or meaning in otherwise unsatisfying existences.

Compulsive use: A patterned behavior of high frequency and high level of intensity, characterized by a high degree of psychological dependence and perhaps physical dependence as well. The distinguishing feature of this behavior is that drug use dominates the individual's existence, and preoccupation with drug taking precludes other social functioning.

Two definitions of "drug abuse" are currently in common use. The social definition, similar to that proposed by Dr. Jaffe, focuses on the drug itself and is the one most often used by law enforcement agencies. The medical definition of drug abuse is "the persistent use of a psychoactive drug that is seriously interfering with an individual's health, economic or social functioning." A medical diagnosis of drug abuse emphasizes chronic, dysfunctional behavior and adverse health consequences and is clinically useful for intervention and treatment of drug dependency problems (Smith & Wesson, 1983).

Addiction is often equated with physical dependence. For a long time, and in keeping with the social definition of abuse, drug abusers have erroneously assumed that if they were not physically dependent on a drug, they were not addicted to that drug. The greatest danger in this notion is that it leads drug addicts to seek detoxification as the sole treatment for their addiction. Also, it exempts addiction to substances that are not illegal.

Looking at addiction as a medical problem and through an extension of the medical definitions of substance abuse, addictionologists—those

health professionals who study and treat drug and alcohol addiction—
have come to adopt the view first advanced by Jellineck in regard to
alcohol. Jellineck proposed that alcoholism is a progressive and potentially fatal disease (Jellineck, 1960).

As an explanation for the addiction to alcohol, a legal drug, this disease concept gained early acceptance and is promoted by Alcoholics
Anonymous (AA), the National Council of Alcoholism, the National Institute on Alcohol Abuse and Alcoholism, and the American Medical
Association (Marlatt, 1983). The extension of the disease concept to
other, illegal drugs is having harder sledding.

The extension of disease concept has come under fire from those who
point out that if addiction is considered a disease, there is an implication
that there are people who can use illegal drugs without fear of consequences—i.e., can jump in the water without getting wet. Along this
same line, it has been argued that drug abusers are let completely off the
hook if they are portrayed as helpless victims of a disease. Further, if
addiction to drugs is a disease, then legislative restriction for those who
do not have the disease becomes harder to justify.

Other critics of the disease model have argued that the concept of addiction as a disease places too much emphasis on medical authority in
determining how society should manage what these critics see as an individual violation of legal, social, or religious norms. Still others feel that
this concept diverts attention from social and economic inequities in our
society.

The disease concept may appear to run counter to many fears that it
excuses drug abuse, but it should be remembered that not all drug abuse
is addiction. Public fear that dangerous drugs may be condoned—even
promoted—can look at alcohol, a legal drug with long-term application
where the disease concept has not lessened penalties for drunk driving or
public intoxication.

While addiction-prone individuals may be genetically helpless to
change their vulnerability, recovery-directed treatment practitioners agree
that these individuals *are* responsible for their own recovery. Further, as it
becomes increasingly possible to ascertain who the at-risk population are,
education in the identification and avoidance of addictive disease is
bound to increase both the individual's sense of responsibility and the
efficacy of prevention.

Addictionologists view addiction as a primary disease entity that can
be manifested through the compulsive use of any of a number of psychoactive substances. There may be a single drug of choice, or there may
be a combination, such as the upper/downer syndromes alternating stimulants with opiate analgesics or sedative-hypnotics.

The disease of addiction appears to have both genetic and sociocultural components. However, people with a genetic predisposition for the disease, which may be indicated by a family history of drug or alcohol addiction, are not foredoomed to a life of addiction. As in other disease processes, the genetically predisposed individual may avoid the complications — in this case — addiction, by avoiding the psychoactive substances that trigger its symptoms.

There is really no way of knowing for sure who is predisposed to addictive disease. There is no addictive "profile." The best clue we have is the evidence that one or both of one's parents, or one's grandparents, had substance abuse problems. People in this category should be warned of their particular vulnerability and counseled on the early signs and symptoms of potential addiction.

The full-blown symptoms of addictive disease are (1) compulsion, (2) loss of control, and (3) continued use in spite of adverse consequences. There are many earlier warning signs — biological indications that a person is in danger of addiction. These signs should be carefully identified and patients counseled about their meaning.

The biological basis of drug hunger and compulsive substance abuse is the human metabolism's adaptation to addictive drugs. These substances have a profound effect on the way the brain sends its messages and gets things done. Repeated use of a psychoactive substance is a way of re-achieving a desired state. These sought-after changes in consciousness vary among addicted individuals and determine an addict's drug of choice.

The human organism, however, strives to maintain a balance. When faced with an overabundance, it will produce enzymes that aid in the metabolization of that substance. Consequently, the user will find that the drug of choice seems to decrease in potency and duration of effect over time. The abuser or the addiction-prone person will react to these increased enzyme levels by increasing the dosage of his or her drug of choice. This phenomenon can be seen not only with street-drug users but with patients on clinical doses of psychoactive drugs as well. Complaints from a patient that the medicine is "no longer working" should be seen as a danger sign that at least physical dependence is developing.

This is tolerance. *Tolerance* refers to (1) the requirement of progressively larger amounts of a substance to achieve its desired effect or (2) a diminished effect with regular use at the same dose. *Physical dependence* is evidenced by withdrawal symptoms that may appear when the individual stops taking the substance.

Besides the onset of tolerance and physical dependence as indicated by withdrawal symptomatology, there are other ways of recognizing addictive disease. Some of the clues are as follows (Smith et al., 1984):

- A pattern of pathological drug abuse manifested by intoxication throughout the day
- Inability to reduce intake or stop use
- Repeated attempts to control use with periods of temporary abstinence or restriction of use to certain times of the day
- Continuation of substance abuse despite a serious physical disorder aggravated by the use of the substance
- The need for regular use of the substance for adequate functioning
- An episode of complication as a result of intoxication (such as alcoholic blackout or opiate overdose).

Compulsive abuse of certain drug groups may produce physical dependence. However, physical dependence is not a prerequisite of addictive disease. For this reason, diagnosis of addiction should focus on behavior and its consequences to the user. These dysfunctions can take many forms, including occupational and social dysfunction; inability to meet important obligations to friends, family and coworkers; erratic, impulsive or aggressive behavior; legal problems. Automobile accidents, home injuries, even frequent illnesses can be signs of addiction.

Early recognition of addictive disease is complicated by the high degree of denial exhibited by its victims. Much of this denial may be the result of cultural stereotypes that picture the drug addict as either a criminal or morally degraded. In many professions, the discovery of addiction can still mean dismissal and loss of livelihood.

Substance abusers are more often open to admitting their problem both to themselves and others if they are not held morally, spiritually, or intellectually responsible for their compulsive patterns of destructive behavior. According to the disease theory of addiction, addicts are not responsible for the symptoms of their disease, but are responsible for their program of recovery. Along with credible diagnosis, a rational intervention approach meets the abuser with a sense of optimism and hope. It is important to stress that recovery is possible and can be a very positive, life-enhancing process.

RECOVERY

Addiction is an incurable disease. No addict can go back to controlled use of the drug of choice or any other psychoactive drug. To do so is to risk a rapid return to a pathological and deteriorating state that if untreated will result in death.

There is, however, remission from this disease. Remission from active addiction is called "recovery" and centers on abstinence from all psychoactive substances.

Going it alone to achieve recovery is not recommended. The common result is "white knuckle sobriety," an undesirable state wherein unresolved stresses and tensions can cause every bit as much damage as the addiction this mental putting on of brakes and gridlock is intended to avoid.

There are, however, many forms of treatment available to the recovering addict. These include individual and group counseling, inpatient treatment, and such self-help groups as Alcoholics Anonymous, Narcotics Anonymous, and Cocaine Anonymous. In fact, there is currently a proliferation of treatment and self-help programs to fit just about any circumstance, social level, or drug of choice the addict may have. These provide that long-term support that the chronic disease of addiction demands for long-term—life-long—abstinence and recovery.

Practitioners are recognizing that there are delayed withdrawal symptoms. These are flareups that may occur months or even years after withdrawal, during which the recovering person is particularly vulnerable to relapse and needs help.

The pathology of addiction usually affects not only the addict but everyone around the addict as well. Programs such as AlAnon address this issue at a self-help level. Sharon Wegscheider-Cruze, long a recognized authority in this field, advocates the involvement of the whole family and close friends in the process of treatment and recovery.

An interesting direction in addiction research is being taken by Kenneth Blum, PhD, at the University of Texas (Blum, 1984). Blum's research involves the locus ceruleus, an area of the brain that produces a hypersympathetic discharge, in conjunction with both psychoactive drug use and the onset of drug hunger, whether produced by a specific drug challenge or by environmental cues. This discharge appears to be controllable with the use of certain amino acids (proteins), the ingestion of which is compatible with the tenets of abstention and recovery. This research may lead to a means of decreasing drug hunger and its resultant stress and danger of relapse among recovering people.

In that addiction and addictive disease are seen as being progressive, the goal in treatment is to diagnose and intervene as early as possible. The earlier addictive disease is diagnosed, the easier it is to treat. For example, early-onset alcoholics respond to treatment better than older long-term patients with such complications as developed addiction pathology and a diseased liver.

Addictionologists are learning that the traditional linkage of addiction with a preexisting character disorder only exists in a small number of cases. Addiction produces its own pathology. There really is no psychiatric profile of addiction. Diagnosis, therefore, is based on family history and early signs of vulnerability to addiction.

Not all abuse is addiction, and the earlier the distinction can be made in a patient the better. Addiction and abuse call for different programs of treatment: for the addict, counseling and education on the disease and abstinence; for the abuser who is not addiction vulnerable, more likely education, counseling, and development of control and responsibility.

In diagnosing the individual who is having alcohol or drug problems, the first place to look is the family history. If at all possible, this should include grandparents. Overt addiction will often skip a generation, with the children of addicts becoming abstainers because of childhood experience living with addicted parents. However, the vulnerability continues even though the immediate parents may have been lifelong abstainers from psychoactive substances.

The other diagnostic clues will be biological and behavioral. The addiction-prone individual does not react to drug and alcohol experimentation the way a nonprone individual does. For example, a group of teenagers have a party and get drunk. Some of them get sick, some of them pass out. One has a five-hour motor-functional blackout. That is not a normal first-time drinking reaction. On checking out the teenager's family medical history clinicians learned that although both parents are teetotalers, one grandparent underwent treatment for alcoholism.

In this particular case, the 16-year-old subject was aware through her parents of the possible vulnerability she had to psychoactive substances. After this one incident, she adopted a drug-free lifestyle and is leading a healthy life. Not all cases are this successful, but the experience does point up the value of early identification and intervention.

Drug Scams:
The Patient Hustler

There are many drug abusers who neither get their supply of psychoactives from an underground street dealer nor steal them. These abusers go directly to the most reputable of sources, the prescribing physician. Such an abuser is known in the trade as the patient hustler, and what these patients do is perpetrate drug scams. The term *drug scam* has come into our terminology from the street and remains the most accurate description for the confidence games drug abusers play to induce physicians to administer or prescribe their drug of choice. The practice of drug scamming is also known as "working" or "making" a doctor. Often scammers will work a territory, going down a list of physicians. They are good at what they do and can be very convincing. No physician's practice is free from the patient hustler. They operate in all neighborhoods, preying on the clinic, hospital private practice, or rural or neighborhood health center. They may appear in a busy emergency room, a ghetto storefront center, or an exclusive treatment center.

In presentations at our Physician Prescribing Practice conferences, John Chappel, MD, has identified four general manipulative approaches that these scammers may use; (1) feigning physical problems, (2) feigning psychological problems, (3) deception, and (4) pressuring the physician.

Feigning Physical Problems. A variety of physical problems can be convincingly portrayed by drug-seeking patients. These run the gamut from bleeding (often simulated by the use of anticoagulants) and self-inflicted skin lesions to gastrointestinal and musculoskeletal disorders. Three of the most common presenting ailments among patients who seek narcotic drugs are renal colic, toothache, and tic douloureux.

The patient feigning renal colic complains of pain on the left side of the body (to avoid a diagnosis of appendicitis) and a burning sensation on urination. If the physician asks for a urine sample, the patient might even prick his finger and drop a little blood into the urine.

Patients presenting with "toothache" often claim to be from another town and to have left at home the medications prescribed by their own dentists. Should the physician wish to verify this claim, the telephone number supplied for the home-town dentist often is that of an accomplice.

If the person actually has an abscessed tooth, he or she usually makes full use of it by visiting a series of physicians and dentists to ask for pain medication.

Tic douloureux is a favorite approach among patient hustlers because it has no clinical or pathological signs. Patients complain of recurring, intense episodes of facial pain lasting several seconds to several minutes. Some patients are able to contort their faces to simulate an attack of pain.

Feigning Psychological Problems. Most drug seekers who feign psychological problems are attempting to obtain stimulants or depressants rather than analgesics. The psychological complaints most often presented include anxiety, insomnia, fatigue, and depression.

Deception. Manipulations employed to deceive physicians include prescription theft, forgery and alterations, concealing or pretending to take medications, and requesting refills in a shorter period of time than originally prescribed (often with the excuse that the medication was lost or stolen).

Pressuring the Physician. Coercive tactics include eliciting sympathy or guilt (as by suggesting that medical treatment caused the patient's drug dependency), direct threats of physical or financial harm, the offer of bribes, or using the names of influential family members or friends.

Patient-manipulators can go to great lengths. In one case, a recovering narcotic abuser later admitted to having undergone a lung operation he knew he did not need in order to assure an ongoing supply of analgesics.

In another case, a vagrant who had been jailed went into opiate withdrawal and was admitted to the county hospital. There, the physician elected to provide methadone on the basis of the patient's inflated description of his habit. Later, the patient complained again of withdrawal, saying that he had understated his habit. He received a higher dose of methadone. Then he "admitted" to a massive sedative-hypnotic habit as well and demanded medication for downer withdrawal. The patient was in abuser heaven. He found he could get anything he asked for from the hospital. But the situation did not last for long. The scammer had actually outsmarted himself by demanding more drugs than his body could handle, and the hospital literally killed him with kindness.

Although the basic scams look pretty transparent when they are down in black and white on paper, in a busy office, an emergency room where the patient load is piling up, or in the confusing presence of a fast-talking scam expert, the situation can be blurred. Chappel points out several patterns of behavior common among drug scammers that an alert physician can look for:

• The patient who presents a dramatic and compelling but vague complaint.

- The patient whose subjective complaints are not accompanied by the usual objective signs.
- The patient who makes a self-diagnosis and specifically requests a certain drug.
- The patient who has no interest in a diagnosis, fails to keep appointments for x-rays, or laboratory tests, or refuses to see another physician for a consulting opinion.
- The patient who rejects all forms of treatment that do not include psychoactive drugs.

Often a physician will be tempted to give manipulators what they want, just to get rid of them. This can be a great mistake. Word can spread in the drug-using population that a certain doctor is an "easy mark." A physician who prescribes out of ignorance, or one who caves in to the demands of manipulative patients may find him- or herself with a patient load that is definitely unwanted.

In states where the prescribing of psychoactive drugs is closely monitored, these physicians may also find themselves with unwanted attention from peer quality control units and law enforcement authorities. Although prescribing-practice surveillance is primarily geared to identifying and prosecuting "script doctors" — those who "sell" prescriptions for psychoactive drugs — the misprescriber is often caught in the net and may be subject to disciplinary action as well.

In California and certain other states, investigating units and boards of medical quality assurance are attempting to define the differences between the misprescriber who through ignorance may make mistakes or fall prey to drug scammers and the script doctor who is a criminal and should be prosecuted. Educational alternatives have been established, such as our own prescribing-practice courses, which are now taught on a regular basis by the state medical association. It is still up to individual practitioners, however, to take steps to guard against their own vulnerability.

In general, physicians should make themselves familiar with the federal and state schedules for psychoactive drugs. They should also understand the indications and abuse potential of any psychoactive medication that they prescribe. They should be aware of the limitations on prescribing, and if they feel that they must exceed them, do so with clear medical reason and consultation when necessary. Full records should be kept.

The American Medical Association, in collaboration with a number of other professional organizations and federal agencies, developed a series of guidelines that all felt constituted "acceptable professional responses to the demands of the Controlled Substances Act." These guidelines were formulated not as a code of ethics or a body of law but as a "supplement

and support to the ethical principles endorsed by the prescribing professions" (Wilford, 1981). We have included them in that interest. There are
six general and eight specific guidelines (see Box).

Box 1:
AMA Guidelines Administering and Prescribing
Controlled Substances

General Guidelines

1. Controlled substances have legitimate clinical usefulness
and the prescriber should not hesitate to consider prescribing
them when they are indicated for the comfort and well-being
of patients.
2. Prescribing controlled substances for legitimate medical
uses requires special caution because of their potential for
abuse and dependence.
3. Good judgment should be exercised in administering and
prescribing controlled substances so that diversion to illicit
uses is avoided and the development of drug dependence is
minimized or prevented.
4. Physicians should guard against contributing to drug
abuse through injudicious prescription writing practices, or by
acquiescing to unwarranted demands by some patients.
5. Each prescriber should examine his or her individual prescribing practices to ensure that all prescription orders for controlled substances are written with caution.
6. Physicians should make a specific effort to ensure that
patients are not obtaining multiple prescription orders from
different prescribers.

Specific Guidelines for Writing Prescriptions

1. The prescription order must be signed by the prescriber
when it is written. The prescriber's name, address, and DEA
registration number as well as the full name and address of the
patient, must be shown on prescriptions for controlled substances.
2. The written prescription order should be precise and dis-
tinctly legible to enhance exact and effective communications
between prescriber and dispenser.
3. The prescription order should indicate whether or not it
may be renewed and, if so, the number of times or the duration

for which renewal is authorized. Prescription orders for drugs on Schedules III, IV, and V may be issued either orally or in writing and may be renewed if so authorized on the prescription order. However, the prescription order may be only renewed up to five times within six months after the date of issue. A written prescription order is required for drugs in Schedule II. The renewing of Schedule II prescription orders is prohibited. A dispenser may accept an oral order for Schedule II drugs only in an emergency, and such an oral order must be followed up by a written order within 72 hours. Controlled substances that are prescribed without an indication for renewal cannot be renewed without authorization by the prescriber.

4. Physicians should prescribe no greater quantity of a controlled substance than is needed until the next check-up.

5. Prescription orders should be made alteration-proof. When prescribing a controlled substance, the actual amount should be written out as well as given in Arabic numbers or Roman numerals to discourage alterations. Prescribers should consider placing a number of check-off boxes on their prescription blanks to show amounts within which the prescribed amount falls, such as 1-25, 26-50, 51-100, and over 100.

6. A separate prescription blank should be used for each controlled substance prescribed.

7. Physicians should avoid using prescription blanks that are preprinted with the name of a proprietary preparation.

8. When institutional prescription blanks are used, the prescriber should print his/her name, address, and DEA registration number on such blanks (Wilford, 1981).

In general, a prescriber is expected to work within the community standards of care, whatever they may be. This may be furthered by attendance at pertinent continuing medical credit courses, reviews of the current literature, and consultation with experts in the field when necessary. All of this may involve time and effort, but it is much better in the long run than making a medical mistake that could have been avoided (Smith & Seymour, 1983).

Continuity of Care:
Program Function and Appropriateness

In the United States, there is a polychromatic spectrum of care available to substance abusers. We feel this variety of treatment is important. There are many variations of response to treatment, and monochromatic, single-treatment approaches have tended to lack effectiveness. On the other hand, those cultures that have accepted the multiple nature of substance abuse and responded to it have profited by their diversity.

Single solutions to substance abuse problems tend to be political. Single solutions are less expensive, easier to control, and easier to promote. They take into consideration the needs of the polis but not the varied needs of the patient. In this chapter, we will review some of the most prevalent treatment modalities and their appropriateness to problem groupings.

METHADONE MAINTENANCE

First proposed in 1964 by Drs. Vincent Dole and Marie Nyswander, methadone maintenance came to be embraced by the U.S. government as a "solution" to the heroin addiction problem. Fortunately, it never did become the sole treatment modality for heroin addiction here as it did in several other countries.

It should be pointed out that prior to the adoption of methadone maintenance, the nationally accepted treatment model for heroin addiction was a form of enforced "cold turkey" provided at such federal prison facilities as Lexington, Kentucky. The government had been looking at the British system of actually providing heroin to its addicts. The British system had its moral drawbacks from the American view, but the Lexington system resulted in a very high rate of relapse as soon as the addicts were released.

Dole and Nyswander, pioneers in the research of addiction treatment, selected methadone as their treatment agent because it was inexpensive, because it was effective when taken orally, thus eliminating the need for injections, and because its length of effect made once-a-day administration on an outpatient basis feasible. Because methadone was a synthetic that called for a highly sophisticated process of synthesis, it was argued that the government could maintain tight control of its production and distribution. A political plus was that tight control could also be kept of the addicts using methadone.

For all its shortcomings, methadone maintenance did seem to provide a more humane way of dealing with opiate addiction than incarceration and restraint. The theory was that methadone maintenance would give addicts a more stable lifestyle and minimize their addiction-related illegal activities. Administered or provided on a daily basis at licensed clinics, methadone would eliminate the pressure for buying heroin or other opiates by preventing opiate withdrawal symptoms and by blocking the euphoric action of these drugs. The dosage could be controlled at a level that would minimize desirable opiate effects but would reduce craving for heroin and other opiates. It would also block and reduce the effect of any opiate the client attempted to inject.

It should be kept in mind that methadone will not work for any drug problems other than opiate problems. It will not block the effects of either sedative-hypnotic drugs such as barbiturates or alcohol or such stimulants as amphetamine and cocaine.

On the plus side, methadone maintenance will provide addicts who have been unable to stay off opiates in any other way and who have exhausted all other treatment opportunities, a means of stabilizing their lives. With regular methadone, they can hold steady jobs that do not involve intricate cerebration or mechanical responsibility. They can be free of the criminal activity needed to support continuous narcotics addiction.

On the minus side, methadone maintenance is essentially trading one addiction, an illegal one, for another that is state approved. Methadone is considered to be a stronger drug than heroin and harder to detoxify. Other considerations involve the availability of maintenance and who is indicated. Many opiate abusers seek treatment after only a short period of abuse while their tolerance has not yet forced a high dose and their addiction is at worst borderline. Maintenance for these abusers may result in a solidification of addiction when their problem might best have been dealt with through some other modality that does not involve the use of narcotics in treatment.

Where methadone maintenance is used, it is usually accompanied by counseling and other treatment. There is some tendency, however, toward just providing maintenance on a daily basis without any attempt to treat the addiction. Physicians referring clients to maintenance programs should check the programs out carefully beforehand and make sure that other necessary services are provided.

METHADONE DETOXIFICATION

In cases of opiate dependency, methadone may be used for substitution and detoxification. This treatment modality is similar in both intent and execution to phenobarbital substitution and withdrawal for sedative-hypnotic drugs. Here, the opiate-dependent individual is given methadone to block withdrawal effects of the opiate, and then the methadone is gradually withdrawn. This procedure is usually accomplished on an outpatient basis. When detoxification is completed, the client is referred into drug-free treatment.

CLONIDINE DETOXIFICATION

Clonidine has been marketed in the United States as Catapres® since 1974. Its primary indication is for the treatment of hypertension. Within the central nervous system, clonidine apparently binds to alpha 2 receptor sites. This inhibits the release of norepinephrine and thereby diminishes central sympathomimetic outflow, producing peripheral vasodilatation and decreased heart rate.

In opiate detoxification, clonidine seems to work on the principle that the opiate withdrawal syndrome is, in part, due to sympathetic hyperactivity. This view is supported by the observation that clonidine will partially block the signs and symptoms of sympathetic hyperactivity in opiate-dependent individuals that are precipitated by the narcotic antagonists naloxone, and naltrexone.

In 1981, John P. Morgan, MD, and Donald R. Wesson, MD, reported on their experimental treatment experience with clonidine as follows.

> They are generally started on 0.1 mg. to 0.2 mg. four or five times per day for 7 days; then the dosage is dropped off, stepwise, over a four-day period. With long-acting opiates such as methadone, the stabilization period is 10 days. To avoid any escalation of the dosage, patients are seen daily and the day's supply of medication is dispensed.
>
> When clonidine is used in this manner, orthostatic hypotension and other side effects have been minimal. A few patients have complained of feeling "spacy" or dysphoric, and some report inadequate symptom relief. Most patients report rapid relief of anxiety, chilling, runny nose, and gastro-intestinal upset, 30 to 60 minutes following an oral dose. Clonidine does not, however, appear to suppress the dull aches in muscles and joints.
>
> Adjunctively to clonidine, we have used L-tryptophan in dosages of 1000 to 3000 mg. per night to assist with sleep, and aceta-

minophen (Tylenol®) in dosages of 1 gram, three times a day, to assist in reduction of bone pain (Morgan & Wesson, 1981).

Although clonidine does not bind to opiate receptor sites, nor does it produce euphoria, it does reduce many of the symptoms of opiate withdrawal. This effect is thought to be due to reduction in sympathomimetic outflow from the central nervous system. The value of clonidine in treatment of narcotic addiction is limited to the relief of symptoms during the detoxification phase, seven to ten days. It is not a drug for maintenance therapy.

AGONIST/ANTAGONIST MAINTENANCE

We have seen an example of agonist maintenance in the discussion of methadone maintenance. In simple terms, agonist maintenance is a means of treatment—*any* means of treatment—that involves the use of one's drug of choice or a drug in the same drug group to indefinitely postpone withdrawal symptomatology. The basic theory, as we have seen with methadone maintenance, is that of controlling rather than eliminating addiction.

Methadone maintenance is currently the only accepted agonist treatment modality in the United States. Some research has been done on the use of propoxyphene (Darvon®) as a methadone-type maintenance drug, but its use was outlawed by international accord in the late 1970s.

Opiate antagonists are drugs that block the opiate-utilized receptor sites so that narcotics have no effect on the user. The primary candidate for opiate and opioid antagonist maintenance is naltrexone. This drug effectively blockades the receptor sites while having no psychoactive effect on the user. It is taken orally, and one dose can provide up to three days protection. Researchers indicate that it may be most useful for highly motivated narcotic addicts who cannot take methadone for professional reasons, such as physicians and those who operate machinery.

NON-NARCOTIC SYMPTOMATIC MEDICATION

Usually operational on an outpatient basis is the daily issuing of medications that deal with the opiate and opioid withdrawal symptomatology on a symptomatic basis. This treatment is usually an adjunct to counseling. The client receives counseling daily during withdrawal, and each day is given one day's worth of medication based on the withdrawal problems that client is currently experiencing. These medications are not narcotics and are not maintenance drugs. If anything, they are usually not very abusable drugs with little or no street value.

RESIDENTIAL TREATMENT

Residential treatment, based on either a social or medical model or some combination of both can be highly effective not only for narcotic detoxification and aftercare but for the treatment of a number of other drug problems as well. In the 1960s and 1970s, most residential treatment was based on the social model and included such programs as New York's Daytop Village, San Francisco's Delancey Street, and the somewhat ubiquitous Synanon. Such programs involved all aspects of the clients' lives and came to be known as "therapeutic communities," or TCs.

Treatment for withdrawal at TCs can range from drug free to full medical substitution. Often, however, reliance for therapy is placed on counseling and group processes in a closely knit "community."

In recent years, many hospitals have established "drug treatment wings" and "chemical dependency units." These usually look to third-party support through employee or individual health insurance and receive referrals from employee assistance programs. Many of these programs are impressively staffed and equipped, but it should be kept in mind that different treatment needs require different modalities. Anyone seeking residential or inpatient treatment for a client should carefully review the available alternatives.

It should be kept in mind that the therapeutic communities have helped many thousands of drug abusers and addicts who would have been considered lost causes in other, more medically directed programs. The real, deep-seated needs of the client should be taken into consideration.

The one negative quality that may appear in a TC, or in any program that works closely with its clients over a long period, is the tendency toward the program's becoming an end in and of itself. In the extreme, this tendency can lead to program's becoming a cult centered on its founder or a charismatic leader. A warning sign can be the program's tendency to hold on to clients and lead them deeper and deeper into the program itself.

A most welcome tendency in nearly all residential treatment programs is the adoption of the disease concept of substance abuse and with it an increasing emphasis on ongoing self-help work and recovery.

SELF-HELP PROGRAMS

Down through the years, Alcoholics Anonymous and other self-help programs have proved to be amont the most effective long-term means of dealing with addiction and recovery. These programs employ the use of twelve steps and frequent meetings in dealing with addiction. Although the steps often mention a "force greater than oneself," they are a combination of pragmatic and spiritual rather than dogmatically religious in their approach to substance addiction. Although originally founded to deal with alcoholism, the twelve-step programs now include programs for narcotic and cocaine users, relatives of alcoholics and other addicts, and overeaters and are beginning to appear in other areas where one encounters compulsive behavior, such as gambling and sex.

OTHER TREATMENT

Sedative-hypnotic withdrawal, including that for alcohol addiction, can be a life-threatening procedure and should be accomplished in an inpatient setting where vital signs can be monitored and such medical emergencies as major seizures can be dealt with quickly. Ordinarily, stimulant, narcotic, and psychedelic withdrawal can be handled on an outpatient basis if there are no complications.

Social complications, especially among the very young, may cail for long-term treatment in a therapeutic setting. Cocaine withdrawal or other instances in which the client is especially vulnerable to drug hunger may call for inpatient time to protect the client from gaining access to more cocaine and relapsing.

Support groups for those recovering from specific drugs, such as cocaine, or in similar work or social situations, such as addicted nurses or doctors, can be very helpful to the recovery process. These programs should be facilitated by professionals familiar with the particular addiction or support population.

Experimental Treatment

First used in Hong Kong and at the Haight-Ashbury Free Medical Clinic as an alternative to symptomatic medication in supervised narcotic withdrawal, acupuncture is proving an effective aid in detoxification from a variety of drug problems. It has also proved useful in the treatment of related health problems that involve compulsive behavior.

Acupuncture has been used in the Orient for thousands of years to treat a wide variety of medical problems. Treatment consists of inserting very thin needles into specific points in the body at the center of areas called *meridians*. These meridians are directly related to internal organs and other parts of the body. Stimulation of a given set of points can have an analgesic effect on whatever organ the meridian is related to. Some practitioners claim a curative and restorative effect as well.

Traditionally, the needles were twirled or jiggled to produce stimulation. Today, most practitioners employ small, low-voltage transformers that send a trickle of electricity through the needles. The current is not painful; it feels like a tiny shower massage. The earliest "needles" were fishbones, bamboo splinters, and pointed stones. Most needles now are made of silver, gold, or stainless steel and are sterilized before each use.

Like much in Eastern medicine, acupuncture has been little understood by Western scientists. Eastern medicine is based on a totally different set of principles than is our own. Even the terms *yin* and *yang* are hard to define in our cosmos, and meridians have no equivalent in Western medicine. Until recently, the effects of acupuncture were written off as placebo reactions — working only through the power of suggestion.

In the mid-1970s, however, this dismissal of effectiveness began to change with the discovery of opiate receptor sites. These are the mechanisms within the central nervous system that interact with opiates. The molecules of heroin and other narcotics fit into the receptors like keys into specialized locks, producing all the effects we relate to pain killers and euphoriants.

Scientists realized that these sites were obviously not designed for opiates — that there must be some equivalent, naturally occurring internal substance. They soon detected and isolated opiatelike analgesic euphoriants that are produced within the body. These internal painkillers, endorphins, used the receptor sites that had been taken over by opiates in narcotic abusers.

Further research involving pain stimulation, acupuncture analgesia, and pain recurrence through the use of naloxone, the blocking agent used to counter morphine and heroin overdose, produced a startling revelation. Acupuncture fights pain by stimulating the production of endorphins. Stimulation of meridians can direct the flow of these chemicals to specific parts of the body.

The treatment procedure developed at the Haight-Ashbury Free Medical Clinic, utilizing acupuncture for narcotic withdrawal, was developed by a Malaysian doctor who had treated opium addiction in China before World War II. It was offered to clients in our Drug Treatment Project on a volunteer basis as an experimental alternative to symptomatic non-narcotic medication. In addition to counseling, each client is given 30-minute sessions of electrostimulated acupuncture as needed on a daily basis. The needles are administered to the "lung" and the "God's door" meridians, located in the ear. These sessions are administered with the client lying down in a quiet room. The rheostat (flow control) on the needles is adjusted to a comfortable trickle of stimulation. The client is encouraged to relax and rest during the session. Effects can include:

- Sedation without sedative drug aftereffects
- Relaxation achieved by control of hypotonicity or hyperactivity of organs
- Functional modifications including control of the full range of symptoms associated with opiate withdrawal

Acupuncture would seem to be effective in treating chronic pain, which is a major underlying cause of opiate abuse and relapse after detoxification. By providing nonnarcotic relief from pain, it can reduce the potential of a patient's return to addiction.

Often, when recovering addicts suffer from conventional medical or dental problems, the prescription of codeine or other analgesics for pain may trigger the old craving for opiates. If acupuncture is used to treat that pain, the risk of relapse is lessened.

It is hoped that acupuncture may improve the pain threshold. Clean narcotic addicts are often highly susceptible to pain, perhaps because their ability to produce endorphins has been reduced by the presence of narcotics in the system. Acupuncture may have a long-term positive effect on pain tolerance by stimulating endorphin production.

Acupuncture also seems to be effective in treating a variety of addiction-related problems other than opiate abuse. It has had some success in curbing tobacco smoking, weight disorders, and the drug hunger that follows cocaine addiction.

OTHER EXPERIMENTAL TREATMENT

The treatment of substance abuse is a rapidly evolving field, and many experimental procedures are being tested. It is to be hoped that these will further our ability to deal with the world tragedy of substance abuse and addiction.

At present, some of these procedures involve work with the stimulation of endorphins and other internal substances. Recent studies have indicated that there are also sedative-hypnotic and stimulant receptor sites. Although some of them have not as yet been identified, there are obviously internal substances that provide all the positive effects that are found in psychoactive drugs. Running and aerobic exercise are among the means being used to provide positive effect through stimulation of these substances and reduction of drug hunger among recovering populations.

Diet and dietary supplementation represents another major area of research. Dr. Ken Blum and others are studying the effects of certain amino acids on parts of the brain that are involved in prompting drug-seeking behavior.

Diseases Related to Substance Abuse

Certain diseases and other medical complications occur as a result of alcohol and drug abuse. Many but not all of these are a result of needle use. In examining these substance abuse-related diseases, we will begin with those that are usually caused by injection of drugs.

ACQUIRED IMMUNE DEFICIENCY SYNDROME (AIDS)

Needle-using drug abusers comprise one of the primary populations at risk for AIDS, a usually fatal viral disease. They account for many of the AIDS cases that have been reported to the national Centers for Disease Control. Homosexuals who are also needle-using drug abusers are doubly at risk according to national epidemiological data.

The incidence of AIDS among needle-using drug abusers seems to depend a great deal upon local use traditions and habits. The highest incidence is reported from New York City, where there is a tradition of needle sharing and where "shooting galleries" attract many addicts who share or rent their "works." As of November, 1984, New York City had reported over 800 out of a total 2686 AIDS victims as being heterosexual or homosexual intravenous drug users. By that same time, San Francisco had reported only 8 out of a total 823 AIDS cases as linked directly to intravenous drug use.

San Francisco heroin abusers share needles, too, but seem to be more conservative in their social usage patterns than their East Coast counterparts. Dr. John Newmeyer, the epidemiologist and research director for the Haight-Ashbury Free Medical Clinic, reports that the San Francisco users have an inclination to keep the same "shooting partners" over a long period of time.

San Francisco also has had some success with a nonjudgmental AIDS educational campaign. The gist of the campaign is: "Users who share their needles or use dirty needles are at risk for contracting AIDS through their drug use. Those who use sterile needles are not." Newmeyer conducted a survey of drug users seeking treatment at the Clinic and found that the threat of AIDS had caused 47 percent of the respondents to change their drug-taking behavior.

It should be remembered that not all needle drug abusers are heroin or other opiate users. A percentage of sedative-hypnotic users and those who use stimulants including cocaine also inject their drugs and are vulnerable to the spread of AIDS. It is not the drug but the way in which it is taken that causes the risk.

Very little is known as yet about AIDS as a disease entity. It appears to be a virus that is usually spread through bodily fluids either sexually or through the blood and other bodily fluids. There is no evidence that close, nonintimate contact with an AIDS victim results in transmission of the disease. No health care worker has developed AIDS as a result of caring for AIDS patients.

The primary effect of the disease is the suppression of the patient's immune system, making the victim susceptible to a variety of diseases, including cancers and respiratory ailments that would normally be dealt with by the body's immune system. The diseases are called "opportunistic infections" because they take advantage of the body's lack of defences and include *Pneumocystis carinii* pneumonia, a parasitic infection of the lungs, and Kaposi's sarcoma, a previously rare form of skin malignancy.

The first reported cases of AIDS in the United States were in 1979 among gay and bisexual men who reported a high number of sexual partners. Since then, AIDS has been diagnosed in heterosexual and homosexual intravenous drug users, in Haitian immigrants of both sexes, in prostitutes and female sex partners of IV drug users, and in hemophiliacs and others who depend on frequent blood transfusions to stay alive. There have also been cases among the children of high-risk populations. In any event, it has become obvious that vulnerability to the disease is not limited to any particular segment of the population.

The following signals have been developed by the Haight-Ashbury Free Medical Clinic AIDS screening unit. If any of these appear, a high-risk person should see a physician:

- A new skin rash or lesion anywhere on the body that persists for more than one or two weeks.
- An unexplained weight loss of greater than 10 pounds that persists for more than a month in a previously healthy person
- Unexplained low-grade fever or night sweats that do not go away after two or three weeks
- Persistent diarrhea
- Unexplained fatigue
- Many swollen lymph glands (around the neck, under the armpits, and in the groin area) that do not go away in two to four weeks in an otherwise healthy person

The danger of infection with AIDS virus can be reduced by using condoms during intercourse.

Shooting Up and Your Health, a brochure published by the Haight-Ashbury Free Medical Clinic in San Francisco, explains the hazards of shooting up drugs and lists symptoms of AIDS, hepatitis B, and endocarditis, a bacterial infection of the heart. In addition to providing medical resources, the brochure recommends the following measures for reducing the risk of disease:

- Don't Inject Drugs! However, if you do:

- Don't Share Needles!

  Sharing drugs can share diseases, too. Obtain your own "works" and don't let anyone else use them.

- Clean Your Works.

  Wash them with alcohol after each use, then leave them to soak in alcohol until the next use.

- Clean Your Skin.

  With alcohol, before injecting.

- Keep Healthy.

  If you are in a weakened state, you are more likely to get a disease. Eat a balanced diet, get enough rest and exercise, and get medical care when you need it.

HEPATITIS AND OTHER LIVER DISORDERS

Although AIDS has gotten more attention in recent years, hepatitis B continues to be the most common medical complication of needle drug use. Unlike AIDS, this disease does not spread only by needle use and sexual intercourse. Until a few years ago, it was thought that hepatitis was neatly divided into types A and B. Type A (infectious hepatitis) was spread in the same ways that most contagious diseases are: food, food preparation, sharing of utensils, incidental contact, and so on. Type B, (serum hepatitis), the more serious of the two, was thought to be spread only by blood contact. We now know that the virus that causes hepatitis B can be spread by biting insects such as mosquitoes, by oral intake of the infectious agent, and possibly by sexual intercourse as well. Current research indicates that some forms of hepatitis spread on an anal/oral progression and recommends washing hands thoroughly after all bowel movements as a means of prophlaxis.

Also, unlike AIDS, hepatitis is usully not fatal if it is detected and treated at an early stage. Symptoms of all forms of hepatitis include fatigue, loss of appetite, pain in the upper abdomen, yellow skin and a yellowish to chartreuse tinge to the sclerae, general itching, dark urine — sometimes the color of Coca-Cola, light-colored feces, and depression. Paranoia and some general mental disorientation may occur. Serum hepatitis (B), infectious hepatitis (A), and some other liver problems may be called jaundice, especially if they cause a yellow pallor to the skin.

Gamma globulin injection can provide short-term immunity to all forms of hepatitis and can reduce the symptoms of serum hepatitis if it is given before the disease matures. There is a gestation period.

Treatment includes bed rest and nutritional support along with the avoidance of alcohol or any other substance that may further irritate the liver. The patient should avoid contact with others and should use separate linens and dishes until the symptoms disappear. Hands should be washed thoroughly following any genital contact.

Nonviral forms of hepatitis like liver disease may be caused by drug impurities or by alcohol abuse. This form is often called "junk" hepatitis and usually manifests in the portal tract of the liver. Chronic disease may involve fibrosis of tissue. The drug abuser with hepatitis is three to four times more likely to have hepatic fibrosis if he or she drinks more than 32 ounces of alcohol a week than the abuser who drinks less than 10 ounces a week.

Cirrhosis (scarring) of the liver is most often caused by chronic alcoholism, although it can also result from poor nutrition, viral hepatitis, or "junk" hepatitis. The symptoms of cirrhosis include jaundice (yellowish skin and eye whites), fatigue, ankle swelling, enlargement of the abdomen, and a full feeling in the right upper abdomen.

Treatment for cirrhosis includes total abstinence from alcohol and any other substance that can cause liver irritation or damage. The aim in treatment is to preserve as much of the undamaged liver as possible.

Fatty liver (steatosis of the liver) is a reversible condition that can follow a cycle of excessive drinking in alcoholism. It can also be a precursor of chronic hepatitis and cirrhosis, however. The most sensitive test for alcoholic liver injury is the gamma glutamyltranspeptidase (GGT) test.

Hepatic (liver) carcinoma is rare, but physicians should be alert to its possibility in substance abusers so that its diagnosis and treatment are accurate and early.

There have been reports of liver necrosis, or tissue death, as a complication of solvent abuse. This is more apt to be an industrial problem, affecting workers who are chronically exposed to solvents in the workplace, rather than a complication of intermittent low-dose use for intoxication.

NEEDLE ABSCESSES
AND OTHER SKIN-RELATED COMPLICATIONS

Sidney Cohen, MD, and Donald M. Gallant, MD, have identified several of the dermatological or skin-related problems that result from drug injection:

1. Needle-track scars are caused by unsterile techniques and the injection of fibrogenic particulate matter.
2. In addition, attempts to sterilize the needle by heating the tip with a match causes the deposit of carbon, which causes mild inflammatory reaction; subsequent repeated injection with such a needle causes tattooing or dark pigmentation at the point of entry of the needle. However, macrophages pick up the carbon, and the tracks become progressively lighter. Although most common on the arms, tracks can be found on almost any part of the body, because abusers realize that the arms are the first area to be checked. Even the penile veins have been used for injection. The subcutaneous scars found on the thighs and arms are due to chronic abscesses.
3. Abscess formation (the most common septic problem) is usually easy to recognize. Repeated injections without cleansing the skin around the injection sites produce infections that are most commonly due to skin flora such as staphylococci and streptococci. Anaerobic infections, however, occur at a much higher rate in the drug user who takes the drug parenterally (by injection). These abscesses may sometimes be recognized by the presence of a foul-smelling discharge, less often by gas formation, and by a bizarre type of cellulitis.
4. This cellulitis (perhaps really a fasciolitis) is characterized by a stony or wooden-hard tenseness, which progresses rapidly on an extremity, and not necessarily in association with a recent needle puncture or an infected site. Cellulitis occurs when sedative-hypnotics are injected subcutaneously. The tissue becomes reddened, hot, painful, and swollen.
5. Another complication in an extremity may be caused by intraarterial injection. Intense pain is usually produced distal to the site of injection. Swelling, cyanosis, and coldness of the extremity indicate the onset of a medical emergency. If this condition is untreated, gangrene of the hands or fingers may develop with consequent loss of these parts (sphaceloderma).
6. Camptodactyly (permanent flexion of the fingers) results from recurrent use of the hand veins for injection. Irreversible contracture of the fingers and lymphedema may result (Cohen & Gallant, 1981).

CARDIOVASCULAR DISEASE

Infective endocarditis is highly prevalent among drug abusers. It should be suspected in any needle-using abuser who shows symptoms of fever of unknown origin, heart murmur, pneumonia, embolic phenomena, or positive blood cultures (especially with *Candida*, *Staphylococcus aureus*, enterococci, or gram-negative organisms). However, fever may be the only indication of endocarditis, even with negative cultures.

Endocarditis is a progressive disease characterized by frequent embolization and severe cardiac valve destruction. For this reason, it is imperative that the condition be screened for and treatment begun as soon as possible. Otherwise, the condition can be fatal.

The disease is thought to be the result of repeated introduction of the infective agents into the blood system, usually from nonsterile "works" and unusual methods of injection. However, injection is not always the cause of endocarditis. Pneumococcal endocarditis is the most common endocardial complication among chronic alcoholics. Pneumococcal meningitis is also very common.

Other cardiac or heart problems include myocardial disease (possibly due to direct toxic effects of certain drugs on the myocardium), blood pressure changes, and cardiac arrythmias. Vascular complications include local changes due to thrombophlebitis, arteritis, arterial occlusion, embolic phenomena, angiothrombotic pulmonary hypertension, and other problems due to traumatic or mycotic aneurysms.

Alcohol cardiomyopathy is the result of the toxic effect of alcohol and acetaldehyde. Beriberi heart disease is a rare complication of thiamine deficiency in malnourished alcoholics. "Beer drinker's heart" is a combination of right-sided failure, hypertension, and pericardial effusion probably caused by either cobalt or lead contamination.

Irregular heart rhythms are found with cannabis, cocaine, hallucinogens, amphetamines, and anticholinergic drugs, all of which accelerate the pulse rate.

Cohen and Gallant (1981) point out that vascular changes due to necrotizing angiitis (polyarteritis) have been demonstrated in intravenous amphetamine abusers (mainly methamphetamine), resulting in cerebrovascular occlusion and intracranial hemorrhage. Many of the solvents cause a sensitization of the heart to catecholamines similar to that seen with volatile anesthetics. This reaction can lead to sudden death if ventricular fibrillation occurs. Phencyclidine (PCP) and amphetamines can produce paroxysmal hypertension, which must be treated vigorously at high doses.

SLEEPING DISORDERS

Sleep and psycoactive substances seem to be inexorably tied to one another. One of the primary uses of sedative drugs, such as barbiturates, is the short-term relief of sleeplessness (insomnia). On the other hand, stimulant drugs have often been used to prevent their users from falling asleep. Drugs may be used in the treatment of sleep disorders, or they may cause sleep disorders. Often, withdrawal from certain drugs will involve sleeping problems as well.

While barbiturates and other sedative drugs may be used as an aid to sleep, their withdrawal will often involve an inability to fall asleep. This is also true of withdrawal from alcohol, heroin, methadone, and other opiates and the benzodiazepines. Because the use of these drugs suppresses REM sleep (dreaming phase), their withdrawal can involve a rebound characterized by vivid dreaming, nightmares, and chaotic sleep patterns.

Conversely, stimulants such as amphetamine are used in the treatment of such sleep disorders as narcolepsy, in which the victim is subject to falling asleep at inappropriate times and inappropriate places. Withdrawal from these drugs often involves long periods of both depression and non-REM sleep.

In general, narcotics and sedative-hypnotics produce sleep, while stimulants and most psychedelic drugs inhibit sleep. There are exceptions to this. Marijuana, for example, while usually classified with the psychedelics, has a distinct sedative quality and is used by some to self-medicate sleeplessness. Coffee and tea can produce a varying degree of stimulation and sleep inhibition in their users, while some users report that tea will actually serve as a sedative when taken in a state of fatigue and will induce sleep.

WEIGHT DISORDERS

Unlike the situation with sleeping disorders, wherein there is a fairly sharp division between the effects of drugs on sleep, virtually all drug abuse seems to result in weight loss rather than weight gain. Withdrawal from most drugs may involve weight gain. This may simply involve a rebound from an underweight state that, in recovery, settles at a healthy balance in keeping with one's bodily structure. In some victims of addictive disease, however, the compulsion of drug abuse may be redirected to food. Overeaters Anonymous (OA) and similar programs treat compulsive eating wth a twelve-step program and view compulsive eating as addictive disease not unlike alcoholism and drug addiction.

Many eating disorders seem similar to substance-abuse problems.

These include not only compulsive eating but its opposite number, compulsive noneating (anorexia nervosa) and bingeing and purging (bulimia).
One of the few remaining medical indications for stimulants is short-term weight control. The compulsive use of stimulants, however, can often result in excessive weight loss.

Many of the complications of substance abuse can be a result of malnutrition. This can be seen with opiate abuse and with alcoholism.

In some situations, including compulsive cigarette smoking and stimulant use, the abuse may continue in part throughout the user's fear of weight gain if the use is terminated.

PSYCHOLOGICAL
AND NEUROLOGICAL COMPLICATIONS

Recent studies indicate that addiction may be a pathological state in and of itself. In most cases, what appears to be underlying psychopathology to substance abuse is actually caused by the abuse and addiction rather than being a cause. This is becoming more apparent as more people undergo long-term treatment and enter into programs of abstinence and recovery. Their experiences run counter to the long-held belief that addiction and abuse are somehow the result of an "addictive personality." Addiction is increasingly coming to be seen as a result of physiological genetic factors and psychosocial conditions.

Aside from the question of which came first, however, there are often psychological complications to substance abuse. A major component of any substance abuse treatment regimen is psychological counseling. There are cases in which abuse is actually an attempt to self-medicate problems. Further, powerful drug experiences, such as those encountered with LSD or PCP, can trigger latent psychoses and lead to long-term problems. Psychological and psychiatric considerations with substance abuse are properly the subject of another book.

In that psychoactive drugs are by definition drugs that affect the central nervous system and have their action through it, many of their direct and indirect effects involve the brain and nervous system. These effects, however, may be further complicated by a variety of neurological sequelae. These can include convulsive seizures, cardiorespiratory arrest accompanied by delayed postanoxic encephalopathy, cerebrovascular accidents with embolic phenomena, agitation, tremors, and hallucinosis, all following opiate overdose. Other opiate-related complications include blindness caused by the use of quinine as a cutting agent, acute transverse myelitis characterized by sudden paraplegia and thoractic sensory levels and caused by severe systemic reactions to the opiate or substances such as quinine or other cutting agents, transcient ischemia, hypersensitivity reaction, or a direct toxic effect of the drug. Peripheral-nerve lesions can be caused by direct injection into a nerve, toxic and allergic reactions, or chronic infection. Acute rhabdomyolysis is characterized by skeletal muscle pain and tenderness, swelling, and weakness within a few hours of intravenous injection.

Parkinson-like paralysis reactions have occurred as a result of impurities in underground meperidine (Demerol) that destroy cells in the substantia nigra region of the brain. (This problem is discussed at length in the text on the drug MPPP.)

Bacterial meningitis and central nervous system abscesses are also known to occur in opiate abusers.

Seizures can result from overdoses of opiates, as well as stimulants, and from such psychedelics as LSD and PCP. Seizures are also a hallmark of sedative-hypnotic withdrawal. The occurrence and treatment for these is covered in depth in the general chapter on sedative-hypnotics.

Long-term alcoholism is known to produce cereberal atrophy, and many other drugs produce a variety of cereberal symptoma that may result from so called "brain damage." Research on recovered addicts and abusers indicates that much symptomatology that has in the past been attributed to permanent brain damage is actually reversible with sobriety, abstention, and long-term recovery.

SEXUAL DYSFUNCTION

The interrelation between drugs and human sexuality is a relatively new area of study, but one that is already showing great relevance as well as much confusion and contradiction. It would appear that many substances alter the human sociosexual response cycle either negatively, positively, or both, and that psychoactive drugs that are used recreationally or medicinally may have a profound effect on human sexuality.

Many researchers have claimed, for example, that heroin addiction not only inhibits sexual performance, but may actually replace it. It has been contended that the rush that results from opiate or stimulant injection takes the place of sexual orgasm for many needle-using abusers.

The effect of specific drugs on sexual potency and performance may vary according to dosage, length of time the drug has been used, the individual reaction, and even the predisposition of the researcher. Cocaine, for example, may be a sensitivity and performance enhancer at first, but often it becomes a dysphoriant with chronic use. The same has been said for other stimulants, such as amphetamines.

Drugs in the sedative-hypnotic group, such as alcohol and the so-called "love drug," methaqualone (Quaalude®), may appear to further sex because of their disinhibitory effects. In reality, they can decrease or eliminate function both over time and large dosages.

In general, chronic use of psychoactive drugs seems to have a deleterious effect on human sexuality.

MISCELLANEOUS DISORDERS

A wide variety of other disorders have been directly or indirectly related to drug and alcohol abuse. Many of these are discussed under the specific drugs or drug groups. Since they are disease entities in their own right, aside from their drug relationship, we will not go into detail beyond pointing out the possible relationship they have with abuse.

Both tetanus and malaria can be spread through needle use. Tetanus is more apt to occur from subcutaneous injection or "skin popping" into fat layers where the infection can develop without blood flow contact or vascularization. Malaria strains are usually introduced into the population by users who have spent time in tropical areas where the disease is prevalent. For example, there was an increase on the West Coast after many users returned from Vietnam. Regular tetanus immunization may guard against the first, and quinine presumably kills the malarial parasites when it is used to cut heroin, as is the practice on the East Coast.

Problems in the lungs often develop from inert materials that are used as cutting agents or buffers and binding agents that are used in drugs that come in pill form. These substances do not dissolve, and their particles may become lodged in the lungs, causing chronic pulmonary fibrosis and foreign-body granulomas. One result of this may be pulmonary hypertension which in turn can cause heart failure.

A wide variety of debilitating lung problems may be at least partially induced by substance abuse. These include chronic uvulitis, pharyngitis, and bronchitis from heavy cannabis smoking; tuberculosis, pneumonia, and reduced immune response with malnourished alcoholics; and aspiration pneumonia and pulmonary edema in opiate and sedative-hypnotic abusers.

The blood (hematopoietic) system can exhibit several disorders both in blood producing cells and in the blood itself. Solvent abuse has been associated with bone marrow depression and consequent anemia. Alcohol also has deleterious effects on the bone marrow, and anemia is frequent when the intake of folic acid is low. Bacteremias may be caused by normal skin flora forced into the system by injection as well as by exotic organisms. These can effect the lymphatic system, causing lymphatic lesions in nodes near the injection sites. Chromosome changes and breakages have been related to a variety of drugs.

Production of hormones—testosterone for example—is also affected by a variety of drugs, and the effect of drugs and alcohol on neurotransmitters in the brain is only now beginning to be understood.

Drug abuse has also been linked to kidney abnormalities and renal failure.

Infections reaching the skeleton can be responsible for such bone diseases as septic arthritides and osteomyelitis, while accidents occurring from the clouding of judgment and consciousness may cripple or even kill. Gangrene can develop from the cutting off of circulation to the extremities and may result in amputation. (The instances of this with the drug DOB are discussed in depth in the writeup on that drug in the text.)

Drugs and Pregnancy

Finally, a few words on drugs and pregnancy. It should be kept in mind that virtually all substances ingested by a pregnant mother pass on to the fetus as well. This is just as true for medically prescribed drugs as it is for illegal and recreational drugs. In general, we advise expectant mothers to avoid all drug use during pregnancy. Further, we advise physicians to use extreme caution in the administering of any drug during pregnancy.

Because many substances also pass into the breast milk, similar caution is advised for nursing mothers and their physicians. Expectant and nursing mothers who question this overall restriction on psychoactive substances should keep in mind that they are manufacturing and nurturing a new baby. It follows that they would want to use only the best of ingredients. Even the "social" drugs should be avoided if at all possible. It is becoming evident that cigarette smoking has an effect on birth weight and fetal development, and the dangers of fetal alcohol syndrome (FAS) are becoming well known.

One notable exception to these general rules is the mother who is a regular abuser of opiates or an opiate addict. Under these circumstances, the fetus is also physically dependent on the opiate the mother is using. Any attempt at stopping opiate use during pregnancy may cause potentially fatal withdrawal symptoms in the fetus. This is also true for women on methadone maintenance. The accepted procedure in such cases is to maintain the mother's opiate intake through pregnancy and then detoxify the baby after birth, when withdrawal symptoms can be managed without their becoming life threatening.

Other than the potential for fetal death, the greatest danger in such cases is that the mother's addiction will go unnoticed and the baby's condition will not be treated. Consequently, the diagnostic role of a physician treating a possibly drug dependent neonate is a critical one. Possible early signs are irritability, hypertonicity, high-pitched shrill cries, and tremors. Other signs include vomiting, hyperactivity, poor food intake, diarrhea, fever, sustained Moro (startle) reflex, and seizures. More general signs include sneezing, respiratory distress, twitching, blueness of skin, yawning, apnea, coryza, tearing, and excessive sweating. Low birth weight is also frequent.

Bibliography

Ayers, William A., C.D.C., Starsiak, Mary Jo, M.S., R.N., Sokolay, Phil, M.S. The Bogus Drug: Three Methyl and Alpha Methyl Fentanyl Sold as China White. *Journal of Psychoactive Drugs*, Vol. 13, No. 1, January/March 1981.

Beck, Jerome E., and Gordon, Dale V. Psilocyban Mushrooms. *Pharm-Chem Newsletter*, Vol. 2, No. 1, January/February 1982.

Becker, Charles E., M.D., Roe, Robert L., M.D., Scott, Robert A., M.D. *Alcohol as a Drug*. Medcom Press, New York, 1974.

Blum, Kenneth, Ph.D. *Handbook of Abusable Drugs*. Gardner Press, Inc., New York, 1984.

Bowen, J. Scott, M.D. Diffuse Vascular Spasm Associated with 4-Bromo-2,5-Dimethoxyamphetamine Ingestion. *Journal of the American Medical Association*, Vol. 249, No. 11, March 1983.

Chilton, W. Scott, Bigwood, Jeremy, and Jensen, Robert E. Psilocin, Bufotenine and Serotonin: Historical and Biosynthetic Observations. *Journal of Psychoactive Drugs*, Vol. 11, No. 1-2, January/June 1979.

Cohen, Sidney, M.D. *The Substance Abuse Problems*. The Haworth Press, New York, 1981.

Cohen, Sidney, M.D., and Gallant, Donald M., M.D. Diagnosis of Drug and Alcohol Abuse. In: *Medical Monograph Series*. Eds.: Buchwald, Charles, Ph.D., Katz, Daniel, Callahan, James F., M.A., Career Teacher Center, State University of New York, Downstate Medical Center, Vol. 1, No. 6, October 1981.

Cohen, Sidney, M.D. Inhalants and Solvents. In: *Youth Drug Abuse*. Eds.: Beschner, G. M., and Friedman, A. S. Lexington Books, Lexington, Massachusetts, 1979.

Delliou, D. Bromo DMA: New Hallucinogenic Drug. *Medical Journal of Australia*, Vol. 1, No. 83, 1980.

Dye, Christina. The Name Game — Street Drugs — New, Exotic, Bizarre. *Street Pharmacology*, Vol. 6, Nos. 11-12, November/December 1983.

Ehrlich, Paul, and McGeehan, Maureen. Cocaine Recovery Support Groups and the Language of Recovery. *Journal of Psychoactive Drugs*, Vol. 17, No. 1, January/March 1985.

Farb, Peter, and Armelagos, George. *Consuming Passions: The Anthropology of Eating*. Washington Square Press, Boston, 1980.

Gay, George R. You've Come a Long Way, Baby! Coke Time for the New American Lady of the Eighties. *Journal of Psychoactive Drugs*, Vol. 13, No. 4, October/December 1981.

Ginzburg, Harold, M.D. *Naltrexone: Its Clinical Utility*. National Institute on Drug Abuse Treatment Research Report, OHHS Publ. No. (ADM) 84-1358, Washington, D.C., 1984.

Goldstein, Avram, M.D, Kaizer, S., and Warren, R. Psychotropic Effects of Caffeine in Man. *Journal of Pharmacology, Experimental Theory*, Vol. 150, 1965.

Grinspoon, Lester, M.D., and Bakalar, James B. *Psychedelic Drugs Reconsidered*. Basic Books, New York, 1979.

Grinspoon, Lester, M.D., and Bakalar, James B. *Cocaine: A Drug and Its Social Evolution*. Basic Books, New York, 1976.

Henderson, Gary, M. D. China White, an Update on Identification and Testing. *The PharmChem Newsletter*, Vol. 11, No. 1, 1982.

Huxley, Aldous. *The Doors of Perception*. Harper & Row, New York, 1954.

Hylin, J. W., and Watson, D. P. Ergoline Alkaloids in Tropical Woodroses. *Science*, Vol. 148, 1965.

Inaba, Darryl, Pharm.D. Popper Uh-Ohs or Uh-Oh Poppers! *Kryptonite Gazette*, Vol. 1, No. 3, September 1974.

Inaba, Darryl, Pharm.D. Snappers, Crackle-ers and Poppers. *Kryptonite Gazette*, Vol. 1, No. 2, August 1974.

Institute of Medicine. *Marijuana and Health*. Ed.: Arnold S. Relman. National Academy Press, Washington, D.C., 1982.

Jellineck, E. M. *The Disease Concept of Alcoholism*. Hillhouse Press, New Brunswick, New Jersey, 1960.

Kleber, Herbert D., M.D. *Trexan (Naltrexone HCL): A Pharmacologic Adjunct for the Detoxified Opiate Addict*. E.D. DuPont de Nemours and Co., Inc., Wilmington, Delaware, 1984.

Loisada, P. V., and Brown, B. L. Clinical Management of Phencyclidine. *Clinical Toxicology*, Vol. 9, 1976.

Ling, Walter, M.D., and Wesson, Donald R., M.D. Naltrexone and Its Use in Treatment of Opiate-Dependent Physicians. *California Society for the Treatment of Alcoholism and Other Drug Dependencies*. October/November 1980.

McCoy, Alfred W. *The Politics of Heroin in Southeast Asia*. Harper & Row, New York, 1972.

Manguerra, Anthony S., Pharm.D., and Freeman, Debra, Pharm.D. Acute Poisoning from the Ingestion of *Nicotiana glauca*. *Journal of Toxicology: Clinical Toxicology*, Vol. 19, No. 8, 1982–1983.

Marder, Leon, M.D. Set Up, Loads, Doors or Four Doors. *California Society for the Treatment of Alcoholism and Other Drug Dependencies NEWS*. October/November 1981.

Marlatt, G. A. The Controlled-Drinking Controversy: A Commentary. *American Psychologist,* October 1983.

Menser, G. *Hallucinogenic and Poisonous Mushroom Field Guide.* And/ Or Press, Berkeley, California, 1977.

Micheaux, Henri. *Miserable Miracle.* City Lights Books, San Francisco, 1956.

Morgan, John P., and Kagan, Doreen V., M.S. *Society and Medication: Conflicting Signals for Prescribers and Patients.* Lexington Books, Lexington, Massachusetts, 1983.

Morgan, John P., and Kagan, Doreen V., M.S. The Dusting of America: The Image of Phencyclidine (PCP) in the Popular Media. In: PCP: Problems and Prevention, Selected Proceedings of the National PCP Conference 1979. Eds.: Smith, D. E., Wesson, D. R., Buxton, M. E., Seymour, R. B., Bishop, M. P., Zerkin, E. L. *Journal of Psychoactive Drugs,* Vol. 12, Nos. 3–4, July/December 1980.

Morgan, John P., M.D., and Kagan, Doreen, V., M.S. Street Amphetamine Quality and the Controlled Substance Act of 1970. *Journal of Psychoactive Drugs,* Vol. 10, No. 4, October/December 1978.

Musto, David. *The American Disease.* Yale University Press, New Haven, Connecticut, 1973.

Naranjo, Claudio. *The Healing Journey.* Ballantine Books, New York, 1975.

National Commission on Marijuana and Drug Abuse. *Drug Use in America: Problem in Perspective.* USGPO, Washington, D.C., 1973.

Nickerson, Mark, Parker, John O., Lowry, Thomas D., and Swenson, Edward W. *Isobutyl Nitrite and Related Compounds.* Pharmex, Ltd., San Francisco, 1979.

Sacramento Wire. Killer Drunk-Driver in Trouble Again. *San Francisco Chronicle,* Friday, April 19, 1985.

Seymour, Richard B., M.A. *MDMA.* Haight-Ashbury Publications, San Francisco, 1986.

Seymour, Richard B., M.A., Gorton, Jacquelyne G., R.N., M.S.C.S., and Smith, David E., M.D. The Client with a Substance Abuse Problem. In: *Practice and Management of Psychiatric Emergency Care* Eds.: Gorton, J. G., and Partridge, R. The C. V. Mosby Company, St. Louis, 1982.

Seymour, Richard B., M.A., and Smith, David E., M.D. *Drug Free: Alternatives to Alcohol and Other Drugs.* Facts on File, New York, 1987.

Seymour, Richard B., M.A., and Smith, David E., M.D. Marijuana, Addictive Disease and Recovery. In: *Drug Use in Society: Proceedings of Marijuana and Health Conference, November 1983.* Ed.: Joanne C. Gampel. Council on Marijuana and Health, Washington, D.C., 1984.

Shawcross, William E. Recreational Use of Ergoline Alkaloids from *Argyreia nervosa. Journal of Psychoactive Drugs*, Vol. 15, No. 4, October/December 1983.

Shulgin, Alexander T. MMDA. *Journal of Psychoactive Drugs*, Vol. 8, No. 4, October/December 1976.

Smith, David E., M.D. Treatment Considerations with Cocaine Abusers. In: *Cocaine: A Second Look*. American Council on Marijuana and Other Psychoactive Drugs, Rockville, Maryland, 1983.

Smith, David E., M.D. A New Prescription Drug Abuse Combination: Glutethimide and Codeine. *California Society for the Treatment of Alcoholism and Other Drug Dependencies NEWS*. October/November 1981.

Smith, David E., M.D. A Clinical Approach to the Treatment of PCP Abuse. In: *PCP (Phencyclidine): Historical and Current Perspectives*. Ed.: Domino, E.F. NPP Books, Ann Arbor, Michigan, 1981.

Smith, David E., M.D. Prescription Drugs and the Alcoholic: The Benzodiazepines — Therapeutic and Dependence Considerations. *Proceedings of the Eisenhower Medical Center*. Eisenhower Medical Center, Winter 1981.

Smith, David E., M.D. Editor's Note. In: PCP: Problems and Prevention, Selected Proceedings of the National PCP Conference 1979. Eds.: Smith, D. E., Wesson, D. R., Buxton, M. E., Seymour, R. B., Bishop, M. P., Zerkin, E. L. *Journal of Psychoactive Drugs*, Vol. 12, Nos. 3–4, July/December 1980.

Smith, David E., M.D. Importance of Gradual Dosage Reduction Following Low Dose Benzodiazepine Therapy. *California Society for the Treatment of Alcoholism and Other Drug Dependencies NEWS*, April 1979.

Smith, David E., M.D., and Gay, George R., M.D. *It's So Good, Don't Even Try It Once: Heroin in Perspective*. Prentice Hall, Englewood Cliffs, New Jersey, 1972.

Smith, David E., M.D., Milkman, Harvey B., and Sunderwirth, Stanley G. Addictive Disease: Concept and Controversy. In: *The Addictions: Multidisciplinary Perspectives and Treatments*. Eds.: Harvey B. Milkman and Howard J. Shaffer. Lexington Books / D.C. Heath and Company, Lexington, Massachusetts, 1984.

Smith, David E., M.D., and Seymour, Richard B., M.A. Dream Becomes Nightmare: Adverse Reactions to LSD. In: LSD in Retrospect. Eds.: Sidney Cohen, M.D., and Stanley Krippner, Ph.D. *Journal of Psychoactive Drugs*. Vol. 17, No. 4, October/December 1985.

Smith, David E., M.D., and Seymour, Richard B., M.A. *The Coke Book*. Berkley Books, New York, 1984.

Smith, David E., M.D. and Seymour, Richard B., M.A. Clinical Perspectives on the Toxicity of Marijuana: 1967-1981. In: *Marijuana and*

Youth: Clinical Observations on Motivation and Learning. National Institute on Drug Abuse, Rockville, Maryland, 1982.

Smith, David E., M.D., and Seymour, Richard B., M.A. The Prescription of Stimulants and Anorectics. *Frequently Prescribed and Abused Drugs*, Vol. 2, No. 1, Brooklyn, July 1980.

Smith, David E., M.D., Seymour, Richard B., M.A., and Morgan, John P., M.D. *The Little Black Pill Book.* Bantam Books, New York, 1983.

Smith, David E., M.D., Wesson, Donald R., M.D., and Seymour, Richard B., M.A. The Abuse of Barbiturates and Other Sedative Hypnotics. In: *Handbook on Drug Abuse.* Eds.: Robert L. DuPont, M.D., Avram Goldstein, M.D., and John M. O'Donnell, Ph.D. National Institute on Drug Abuse and White House Office on Drug Abuse Policy, Washington, D.C., 1979.

Smith, David E., M.D., and Wesson, Donald R., M.D. Substance Abuse in Industry: Identification, Intervention, Treatment and Prevention. In: *Substance Abuse in the Workplace.* Eds.: David E. Smith, M.D., Donald R. Wesson, M.D., E. Leif Zerkin, and Jeffrey H. Novey. Haight-Ashbury Publications, San Francisco, 1985.

Smith, David E., M.D., and Wesson, Donald R., M.D. *Treatment of Adverse Reactions to Sedative-Hypnotics.* U.S. Government Printing Office, Washington, D.C., 1974.

Smith, David E., M.D., and Wesson, Donald R., M.D. *Uppers and Downers.* Prentice-Hall, Englewood Cliffs, New Jersey, 1973.

Smith, David E., M.D., Wesson, Donald R., M.D., Buxton, Millicent E., Seymour, Richard B., M.A., Ungerleider, J. Thomas, M.D., Morgan, John P., M.D., Mandell, Arnold J., M.D., and Jara, Gail. *Amphetamine Use, Misuse and Abuse: Proceedings of the National Amphetamine Conference, 1978.* G. K. Hall, Boston, 1979.

Stamets, Paul. *Psilocybe Mushrooms and Their Allies.* Homestead Book Company, Seattle, 1978.

Turek, I. S., Soskin, R. A., and Kurland, A. A. Methylenedioxyamphetamine (MDA): Subjective Effects. *Journal of Psychoactive Drugs*, Vol. 6, No 1, January/March 1974.

Unger, Kathleen Bell, M.D. Methadone in the Relief of Pain. *California Society for the Treatment of Alcoholism and Other Drug Dependencies NEWS*, April 1984.

Wasson, R. Gordon. The Divine Mushroom of Immortality. In: *Flesh of the Gods* Ed.: Furst, P. T. Praeger, New York, 1972.

Weil, Andrew T., M.D. *The Marriage of the Sun and Moon.* Houghton-Mifflin, Boston, 1981.

Weil, Andrew T., M.D. Nutmeg as a Psychoactive Drug. *Journal of Psychoactive Drugs*, Vol. 3, No. 2, Spring 1971.

Weil, Andrew T., M.D., and Rosen, Winifred. *Chocolate to Morphine.* Houghton-Mifflin, Boston, 1983.

Wesson, Donald R., M.D. Naltrexone Approved by AMA. *California Society for the Treatment of Alcoholism and Other Drug Dependencies NEWS.* December 1984.

Wesson, Donald R., M.D., and Smith, David E., M.D. Low Dose Benzodiazepine Withdrawal Syndrome: Receptor Site Mediated. *California Society for the Treatment of Alcoholism and Other Drug Dependencies NEWS.* January/February 1982.

Wesson, Donald R., M.D., and Smith, David E., M.D. *Barbiturates: Their Use, Misuse and Abuse.* Human Sciences Press, New York, 1977.

Whitfield, Charles, M.D. "Xanthines." Unpublished manuscript.

Wilford, Bonnie Baird. *Drug Abuse: A Guide for the Primary Care Physician.* American Medical Association, Chicago, 1981.

Wineck, C. L. A Death due to 4-Bromo-2,5-Dimethoxyamphetamine. *Clinical Toxicology,* Vol. 283, 1970.

Index to Street Names

Poor man's acid (morning glory) 106
Poppers (nitrites) 39
Quackers (methaqualone) 48
Quads (methaqualone) 48
Quas (methaqualone) 48
Reds (barbiturates) 42
Reefer (marijuana) 91
Rock (cocaine) 71
Rufus (heroin) 20
Rush (nitrites) 39
Sandoz (LSD) 98
Scag (heroin) 12
Setups (glutethimide & codeine) 55,125
714s (methaqualone) 48
She (cocaine) 71
Shermans, sherms (phencyclidine) 110
Shrooms (psilocybin) 114
Sinsemilla (cannabis) 91
Smack (heroin) 12
Smoke (cannabis) 91
Snappers (nitrites) 39
Soapers (methaqualone) 48
Sopes (methaqualone) 48
Southwest Asian (heroin) 20
Space caps (LSD) 98

Speed (amphetamine) 63
Speedball (upper & downer) 129
Stofa (heroin) 12
Stuff (heroin) 12
Sunshine (LSD) 98
Synthetic heroin (MPPP) 18 (alpha methyl
    fentanyl) 10
Ts and Blues, Ts & Bs, etc. (talwin &
    tripelennamine) 127
Tiles (DOB) 95
Tonanacatl (psilocybin) 114
Tops & Bottoms (talwin & tripelennamine)
    127
Uppers (amphetamine) 63
Vapors (cocaine) 74
Viper (cocaine) 74
Vitamin V (benzodiazepines) 45
Weed (cannabis) 91
West Coast (methylphenidate Hcl) 80
White crosses (amphetamine) 63
White lightning (alcohol) 36
White lightning [Owsley] (LSD) 98
White pipe (cocaine) 74
Windowpane (LSD) 98
XTC (meth amph) 103
Yellow jackets (Barbiturates) 42

Product Name Index

Quaalude 35,48
Ritalin 80
Robam 55
Robese 63
Rolathimide 55
Rush 39
SK-Bamate 55
Saronil 55
Seconal 42
Sedabamate 55
Serax 35,45
Sernylan 110
Sopor 48

Spancap 63
Stadol 25
Talwin 6,24,127
Tenuate 82
Tidex 63
Tranmep 55
Tranxene 35,45
Trexan 121
Tybatran 55
Tylox 24
Valium 35,45
Xanax 45
Zactane 6

Generic Drug Index

Note: Boldface type denotes page number of sections.

General Index

Drug Related Disease